The Vital
Nerves

The Vital Nerves

A Practical Guide for Physical Therapists

John Gibbons

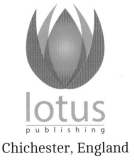

lotus
p u b l i s h i n g

Chichester, England

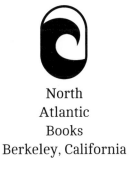

North
Atlantic
Books
Berkeley, California

First published in 2020 by
Lotus Publishing
Apple Tree Cottage, Inlands Road, Nutbourne, Chichester, PO18 8RJ, and
North Atlantic Books
Berkeley, California

Illustrations Amanda Williams
Photographs Ian Taylor
Text Design Medlar Publishing Solutions Pvt Ltd., India
Cover Design Chris Fulcher
Printed and Bound in Malaysia by Tien Wah Press

The Vital Nerves: A Practical Guide for Physical Therapists is sponsored and published by the Society for the Study of Native Arts and Sciences (dba North Atlantic Books), an educational nonprofit based in Berkeley, California, that collaborates with partners to develop cross-cultural perspectives; nurture holistic views of art, science, the humanities, and healing; and seed personal and global transformation by publishing work on the relationship of body, spirit, and nature.

North Atlantic Books' publications are available through most bookstores. For further information, visit our website at www.northatlanticbooks.com or call 800-733-3000.

Medical Disclaimer
The following information is intended for general information purposes only. Individuals should always consult their health care provider before administering any suggestions made in this book. Any application of the material set forth in the following pages is at the reader's discretion and is his or her sole responsibility.

British Library Cataloging-in-Publication Data
A CIP record for this book is available from the British Library
ISBN 978 1 913088 18 7 (Lotus Publishing)
ISBN 978 1 62317 560 3 (North Atlantic Books)

Library of Congress Cataloging-in-Publication Data
Names: Gibbons, John, 1968- author.
Title: The vital nerves : a practical guide for physical
   therapists / John Gibbons.
Description: Nutbourne, Chichester : Lotus Publishing ; Berkeley,
   California : North Atlantic Books, 2021. | Includes bibliographical
   references and index. | Summary: "A must-have book for
   understanding one of the most fundamental areas of physical
   therapy: the nervous system and its relationship to musculoskeletal
   pain"—Provided by publisher.
Identifiers: LCCN 2020012594 (print) | LCCN 2020012595 (ebook) |
   ISBN 9781623175603 (trade paperback) | ISBN 9781623175610 (ebook)
Subjects: LCSH: Nerves, Peripheral—Handbooks, manuals, etc. |
   Physical therapy—Handbooks, manuals, etc.
Classification: LCC QP365.5 .G53 2021 (print) | LCC QP365.5 (ebook) |
   DDC 612.8/1—dc23
LC record available at https://lccn.loc.gov/2020012594
LC ebook record available at https://lccn.loc.gov/2020012595

Dedication

To all the students I have ever taught—without you, none of what I do would be possible, and for that I want to truly thank you!

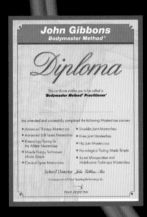
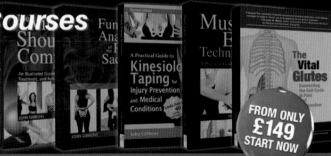

Contents

Acknowledgments

Jon Hutchings—Publisher: I like to think that the professional relationship I have with my publisher, Jon Hutchings, is going from strength to strength. After writing for many years, I still feel honored to have the privilege of being asked again to continue my dream of writing and influencing therapists throughout the world. Without your input and guidance, none of this would be achievable, and I truly thank you for allowing me that opportunity.

Ian Taylor—Photographer: Ian has become a good friend over the years, and with my hand on my heart I honestly believe he completely understands what being an outstanding photographer is all about. He achieves amazing results with the photos he takes because he is a true professional, and it's all about the finer details to get the best results.

Amanda Williams—Illustrator: I reckon I must give my medical illustrator a headache every so often, especially at certain times of the year when I am in constant contact with her regarding the illustrations. I'm sure she doesn't know exactly what it is I want to be drawn sometimes, as I can be a bit vague… I hope that, after many years of being involved with the way I work, she now understands me. I must say, Amanda, you are an amazing medical illustrator, and I truly thank you for all of your hard work.

Stephen Brierley—Editor: Thank you to Steve, who has done an exceptional job yet again of editing this book. He has done a few of my books in the past, and I personally like the way he edits them. Steve is very methodical and precise in his work ethic—thanks for trying your best by modifying and improving my Welsh grammar.

Denise Thomas: Denise has been the model for all of the books to date, which is brilliant, as it shows consistency. She is also my partner (and has been for many years) and especially tolerant of my being grumpy and not particularly nice to be around. I applaud you for sticking with me through the recent difficult times and for being by my side for all these years.

Lee Thomas: Thanks a million to Lee, who has been instrumental in the filming and editing of all the educational videos that are linked via QR codes in this book. You are a true professional in your field and for that I genuinely thank you.

Margaret Gibbons and family: To my mother, Margaret Gibbons—thank you for being there when I have needed you in my life. I wish you all the best and good health in the forthcoming years. I also extend my wishes for a happy and prosperous life to my sister, Amanda Williams, who is approaching 50, to her husband, Philip, and to her son, James, and daughter, Victoria, who are both doing exceptionally well at university and just starting out on their own career pathways.

Lastly, I wanted to say that not a day goes by without thinking about my son, Thomas Rhys Gibbons, who left my world on February 28th, 2017. I would like to think he is looking down on me, feeling proud of what his dad has achieved in his life and knowing that he is changing lives throughout the world. I miss you so much, Tom-Tom—one day, we will be together again.

Introduction

In a nutshell, the neurological testing course at which I lecture at the University of Oxford is, by a considerable margin, the most undersubscribed of all the courses that I currently offer, and this appertains to all the individual practitioners of manual therapy, such as osteopaths, chiropractors, physiotherapists, sports therapists, and even medical doctors. I am not sure why this is, as I always put forward to my students the following statement: out of all of the courses at which I lecture, I feel that the subject area of the nerves and their relationship to the musculoskeletal system is by far the most vital and rewarding. Hence the name of this book.

Nevertheless, basically no matter what I say and what I do in terms of promotion for the course, the attendance is still poor. In reality, I think the reason is because of the words "nerves," "nerve testing," or "neurological." Moreover, whenever I mention to therapists that I am lecturing this particular subject, most of them have the familiar bewildered expression on their faces and answer along the lines of "that's a difficult subject" or "mmm… maybe next time for that course, as it sounds pretty intense."

In terms of my style of writing, I would consider that I have a simple goal, which basically has been applicable to every book I have written to date (or am currently writing)—to try to simplify complex subjects which are related to the anatomy and function of the human body. This process is definitely not as easy as it sounds, and is actually quite a difficult task to undertake, because I too am continually learning and slowly topping up my anatomical base knowledge, within the structure that I personally call my *brain tank*.

I try to improve my ever-expanding tank of knowledge through many different avenues, one of which is attending sports medicine courses; I find listening to surgeons talk about their experiences to be fascinating and truly special. I also spend a lot of time reading and researching material that has been written by world-renowned authors, as well as numerous upon numerous hours researching websites. Doing all of the latter naturally makes me want to write even more about the subject, and therein lies the dilemma. I personally believe that in order to keep the subject matter simple, it has to be written in a simple way; if you know a lot about a subject, then you will of course want to try to write down all the information, plus all the extra bits you research, etc., and suddenly the book becomes unrealistic in terms of the size and content, and needless to say the cost!

When I started on my first book back in 2011, I found writing it to be pretty difficult, as I had never done anything like that before. It was therefore a huge undertaking for me, but eventually the book on muscle energy techniques (METs) was finally published. Even to this day, therapists often comment on "how easy" the MET book is to read, and interestingly the sales of my first book still outsell all of my other books put together.

The reason why I believe my first book is more popular than all of my others is probably because I did not listen to myself when I started to write the second and third books and so on—I should have kept telling myself over and over again, "Keep things simple … keep things simple …" This was especially true when I wrote a book on the pelvis, lumbar spine, and sacroiliac joint, as I am sure you are aware that these areas of the body are most definitely a complex subject. It took over two years for that book to be published, but I must say I am very happy with the outcome. Although people all over the world compliment me on writing such a great book, not once has anybody mentioned to me and commented on "how easy" it was to read!

I do hope that, when therapists read this particular book on the vital nerves, as well as the other components of the nervous system I have included, they will be satisfied that I have been able to at least simplify a complex subject so much so that they (and all readers alike) might actually understand some of the content and, more importantly, enjoy a little of what they have read. If I accomplish any of this to some degree, then I personally believe I have achieved my goal.

This book has not been written with neurosurgeons or neurologists in mind, as I wanted to write it mainly for therapists involved in physical therapy; however, that said, medical doctors should find this text book of interest, because of the detailed explanations and colorful modern images. In reality, we all have to start our careers on the bottom rung of the "learning ladder" no matter where we start out in life, and naturally progress upward from there. My good friend Howard regularly says to me that "every journey starts with a single step, no matter how far you are walking"; this is so true about the subject matter of this book, because sometimes the simple journeys in life are the most rewarding.

Some of the inspiration to write this particular book on the nerves actually came from one of my patients (see the Case Study below)—I found this person's story so fascinating that I thought I would share it with you. By the way, throughout the chapters of this book you will find numerous case studies of actual patients who have visited my clinic at the University of Oxford. I hope that reading about these patients will be of as much interest to you as treating and subsequently writing about them was to me. I believe that writing about individual case studies makes the book far more interesting, especially when the discussion concerns real-life patients who have had some form of neurological disorder. I also hope that reading these unique case histories will have the effect of getting your mind to work like a detective, where you are presented with clues (symptoms); then, through a process of elimination, you can try to solve the mystery (diagnosis/hypothesis of the underlying neurological condition).

Remember, we are all unique individuals. This means that all of us will be at various levels in terms of our own medical knowledge, and naturally we all have different ways of retaining the knowledge that is presented to us. For the reader, I truly hope that this book has the potential to provide at least something that you are able to retain and, more importantly, use in your own career pathway or clinical setting.

CASE STUDY

One of my patients came to see me with a neurological issue with his neck and shoulder. The history of the story was that a year or so prior to seeing me, he was cycling one Saturday morning near his home town and was unfortunately hit by a truck; subsequently, the vehicle actually ended up driving over his torso as well as over his shoulder, with the truck leaving an actual tire mark over his right shoulder region. An ambulance arrived and took him straight to hospital, where he went through the usual examinations of X-rays and MRI scans. Miraculously, he had no fractures or life-threating issues, and was told he simply had some minor nerve damage.

However, especially as time progressed, it became obvious that the injuries sustained were not minor, as he struggled in particular to lift his right arm; he felt very weak and was unable to perform the motion. Nerve conduction studies demonstrated that part of the suprascapular nerve (covered later in this book) was unable to function, with a second MRI showing that the nerve was completely torn from the brachial plexus; the surgeon was not sure if this nerve would regenerate itself. The suprascapular nerve innervates the supraspinatus in its activation, as well as the infraspinatus muscles (these two muscles are part of the rotator cuff group in the shoulder complex), so you can imagine the consequences for the fine-tuning motion of his shoulder if this nerve was unable to regenerate itself.

I saw this patient approximately a year after his accident, when he attended my nerve-testing course with his personal physiotherapist, because they were very interested in trying some different rehabilitation procedures. Basically, when I saw him on the course, he had limited abduction and very weak lateral rotation of the shoulder—it was very obvious (to me) that the muscles (especially the infraspinatus) had atrophied (wasted away). I truly believe that the body is amazing and adapts very well, even in extreme circumstances, because when I asked the patient to externally rotate the shoulder, the teres minor and posterior deltoid "popped" out as if they were on "stage," simply taking the role of the "absent" infraspinatus. Think about this for a moment… These two muscles (teres minor and deltoid) are innervated by a separate nerve called the *axillary nerve* and not by the suprascapular nerve, so basically these two muscles were now providing the motion of external rotation because the infraspinatus was unable to do so. I think this a marvelous feat of ingenuity by the human body.

I advised the patient that I did not believe the nerve would fully regenerate, and remarkably (with the constant help of his physiotherapist) the patient had somehow regained a lot of his lost motion; however, the strength of the movements with the use of a small weight was still obviously weaker, and I said that hopefully, over time, things could improve a bit more.

This particular case study resonated in my mind for many years, and it taught me that the body will try anything to assist and adapt itself to improve. What the case study also demonstrated to me was that I did not possess the skills to actually *fix* his nerve problem—I was only able to advise. For the students attending the nerve-testing course the day he attended, it would have been a great learning curve (hopefully!).

I often smile to myself when I reread that particular case study, as I had just finished writing my previous book— *The Vital Shoulder Complex*—and was starting to write this book actually on the plane traveling to Vietnam for a short holiday. I had literally just finished lecturing a seminar in Taipei, Taiwan and was then off to China to continue my lecturing, before heading back to the UK. My life at the time seemed to consist of traveling to exotic locations, lecturing, or writing, and for that I was truly grateful; I can think of worse ways to spend one's life…!

Within this book, my plan is to mainly focus on the peripheral nervous system (PNS)—what it is all about and how the physical therapist can assess and understand this fascinating area using specialized testing and specific tools, for example a patella or reflex hammer, a tuning fork, or other medical implements. I will not, however, be discussing in depth the cranial nerves (although I will briefly mention them and list them in a table); neither do I plan to spend too much time talking about neurological anatomy and in particular the central nervous system (CNS). That said, although I have written quite a lot about the anatomy and physiology of the nervous system, my attention has been in particular on the PNS, because I wanted the overall focus of the book to be on the fundamentals of how each of these individual systems works. This is through personal choice—I could easily have written about the other subject components, but I consider there to be numerous books on the subject matter (cranial nerves in particular) already. So, why reinvent the wheel and discuss things that have already been adequately covered many times before?

No doubt extra knowledge about neurological anatomy will have its place in the physical therapist's tool box; however, I have been a sports osteopath for many years now and not once (and this is since finishing my osteopathy degree in 2003) have I used the practical skills of cranial nerve examination that all my fellow osteopaths and myself spent many years acquiring. Once this book has been published, if I get asked on a regular basis "Why didn't you include the cranial nerves?" and "Why didn't you add this or that?" for example, might I consider writing a second edition incorporating these additional topics. Until then you will have to consult other books on the cranial nerves and the central nervous system!

A few student osteopaths from the UK used to ask me when my book on nerves was coming out, and I would always say to them: "It will be ready when it's ready, as my book on the shoulder complex has just been released, and most of my previous books have taken between one and two years to complete." It's not that I am slow at writing; it's because of the number of other people involved in the process of getting the book to the shelves so that people can buy it. That's the main reason why it takes so long, and that's just the way it is, especially if you aim to publish a decent book that people make nice comments about. If I am honest, though, I am actually planning on getting this book on the shelf a lot sooner—why? Maybe it's because I am getting used to the whole process of what is expected from me and what I expect from others, and because this is my seventh book to date; so, on paper (at least), it should just be a formality (time will tell, but I doubt it).

I recently read a book called *Do No Harm* by Henry Marsh, a retired neurosurgeon. I found the book fascinating, as each chapter is written about the actual patients he has treated, some with success but sadly some with not so much. His knowledge of neurology and obviously anatomy of the brain, in particular, is exceptional; however, the book was actually fairly easy to read and very enjoyable, as I believe he wrote it in a way that the reader understood (mostly). If I am honest with myself, I am trying to do the same thing with my book, since the subject matter is quite difficult. There is one particular snippet from Marsh's book that made me smile; it takes place when he is operating on the brain, and he says that the patients are normally awake and actually feel "no pain" from his operating procedures. Why, I hear some of you ask? It's because "in order to feel pain in the brain, the brain would need another brain to feel the pain" … quite simple really, when you think about it!

I wish you all the best, and I truly hope (with my hand on my heart) that you enjoy reading this book.

John Gibbons, 2020

List of Abbreviations

ACh	acetylcholine		LOAF	lateral lumbricals (first and second), opponens pollicis, abductor pollicis brevis, flexor pollicis brevis
ANS	autonomic nervous system			
AROM	active range of motion		LT	light touch
ASIS	anterior superior iliac spine		MCP	metacarpophalangeal
CES	cauda equina syndrome		MET	muscle energy technique
CN	cranial nerve		MND	motor neuron disease
CNS	central nervous system		MRI	magnetic resonance imaging
CSF	cerebrospinal fluid		MS	multiple sclerosis
CSP	cervical spine		NHS	UK National Health Service
CT	computed tomography		NSAID	nonsteroidal anti-inflammatory drug
CTJ	cervical thoracic junction		NTT	nerve tension test
CTS	carpal tunnel syndrome		OA	osteoarthritis
DDD	degenerative disc disease		OAF	opponens pollicis, abductor pollicis brevis, flexor pollicis brevis
DRG	dorsal root ganglion			
DTR	deep tendon reflex		PROM	passive range of motion
ECG	electrocardiogram		PD	Parkinson's disease
EDL	extensor digitorum longus		PID	prolapsed intervertebral disc
EHL	extensor hallucis longus		PNS	peripheral nervous System
EMG	electromyography		POP	plaster of Paris
FDP	flexor digitorum profundus		PSA	prostate specific antigen
FDS	flexor digitorum superficialis		PSNS	parasympathetic nervous system
FPL	flexor pollicis longus		PVD	peripheral vascular disease
Gmax	gluteus maximus		RMP	resting membrane potential
Gmed	gluteus medius		ROM	range of motion
Gmin	gluteus minimus		SLR	straight leg raise
HVT	high-velocity thrust		SNS	sympathetic nervous system
IP	interphalangeal		TFL	tensor fasciae latae
JPS	joint position sense		TOS	thoracic outlet syndrome
KISS	keep it simple stupid		ULTT	upper limb tension test
LMN	lower motor neuron		UMN	upper motor neuron

1

Functional Anatomy of the Nervous System

As far back as I can remember, I have always been fascinated with nerves, especially after seeing the plasticized bodies from the Bodyworks exhibition, where one particular cadaver stood out from all the rest because that specimen had all of the nerves exposed. When you are able to see something as fascinating, even exhilarating, as that, you then come to realize just how complex the body is. What I saw on show that particular day was "only" the nerves—no blood or lymph vessels (which would be just as impressive)—simply the nervous system in all its glory (Figure 1.1).

In the past I have always found basic neurological anatomy and physiology a bit boring and rather dull, especially during lectures for my osteopathy degree at university. Neurologists or neurosurgeons typically taught these seminars, and the problem was that even the teacher's *basic* knowledge of neurology was way too daunting and quite possibly overpowering for my fellow colleagues and me. Within a few minutes of sitting in the lectures and listening to these knowledgeable academics I wanted to leave, as I simply struggled to understand anything that was being said and I had no chance of being able to assimilate any of these words into my brain. Even at home or in the library I found it very difficult to read books on the subject of neurology, especially if they were written by academics (and sadly most of the books are written by neurologists, Ph.D. doctors, or surgeons).

It makes sense to start somewhere, and if you are new to this field then I do hope, with my hand on my heart, that I make the subject of neurology a bit more interesting and even more exciting than it was when first taught to me.

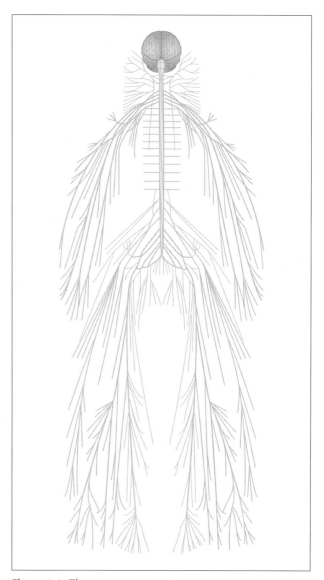

Figure 1.1: *The nervous system in its entirety.*

Nervous System

In simple terms, the nervous system is designed to control the body by sending messages or electrical signals from one part of the body to another, or from one cell to another cell. I consider this system to be the king, queen, or perhaps the president of the country; in other words, it is the ruler, with complete control of everything, and all other systems will bow down to the ruler. This is the role of the nervous system: it is the control center within the human body. All activities within your body, all the organs, all the billions of individual cells, all the physiological and psychological reactions, and all the thoughts are controlled by the nervous system; we cannot underestimate its power. It is considered that approximately 25% of the calories you take in each day are consumed by your brain's activity alone.

In general, the nervous system performs three relatively simple principle functions:

1. *Sensory input* (this information comes in, for example, from the skin or the eyes).
2. *Integration* of the sensory messages (decisions are made at this level).
3. *A motor output response* (i.e., the messages are sent on to another source, such as the skeletal muscles).

Within the human body, the nervous system is made up of two main component systems—the central nervous system and the peripheral nervous system. The *central nervous system* (CNS) is formed from just the brain and the spinal cord, and is the main control center. The *peripheral nervous system* (PNS) is formed from thousands of nerves that link the spinal cord (part of the CNS) to the skeletal muscles as well as to the sensory receptors; this unique system is therefore basically the communication center.

The PNS is subdivided into the *sensory* (afferent) and *motor* (efferent) divisions. The motor component is then subdivided again into the *somatic nervous system* (voluntary system) and the *autonomic nervous system* (ANS—involuntary system). The ANS is further subdivided into what is known as the *sympathetic nervous system* (fight-or-flight response) and the *parasympathetic nervous system* (rest and digest response). These various components of the nervous system are outlined in the flow chart in Figure 1.2.

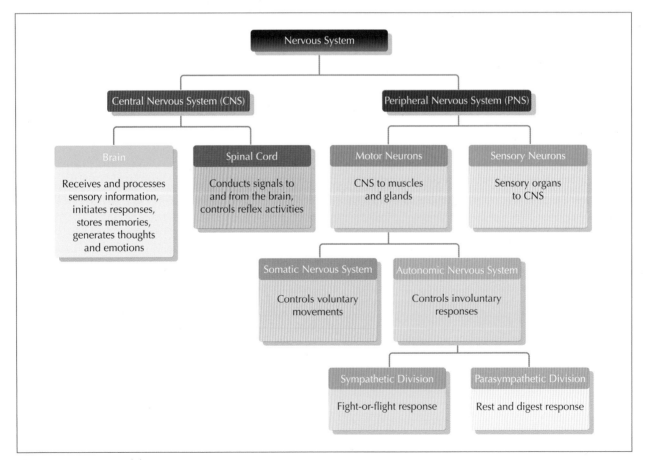

Figure 1.2: *Divisions of the nervous system.*

What is a Nerve Versus a Neuron?

A nerve and a neuron seem to be one and the same to the majority of people, but they are in fact two different structures. The two, however, are naturally linked together, as nerves can be thought of as projections of neurons.

Neurons

Neurons, also known as *neurones* or *nerve cells*, are found within the brain, spinal cord, and peripheral nerves. Neurons are the fundamental units that control everything we do as human beings: they send and receive signals and conduct the signal (the train station), while nerves transmit the information to all parts of the body (the train traveling along the tracks). The brain is thought to have 85–100 billion neurons (*wow!*).

Nervous tissue is basically comprised of neurons, but also has supporting cells that are interlinked to it. These supporting cell structures are known as *glial cells* (also called *neuroglia*) and they make up a high abundance of the cells within the brain (see "Glial Cells" below).

Types of Neuron

Neurons typically share the same structure and are the cells that make up the nervous tissue. A *neuron* has three main parts, as shown in Figure 1.3: a cell body or soma (tree trunk), an axon (tree root), and dendrites (tree branches with associated dendritic spines).

Simply put, the *cell body* is the control center and contains the nucleus and the mitochondria as well as other components. *Dendrites* are the listeners as they are the link in receiving signals and messages from other cells (input); they receive the information via small protrusions called *dendritic spines*, which project from the branches at specialized junction points called *synapses*. The *axon* is basically the talker, and comes into play when a neuron wants to talk to another neuron (the output); it does this through an action potential (all will be revealed later).

Just to complicate matters, there are actually four different types of neuron (Figure 1.4). These are classified as:

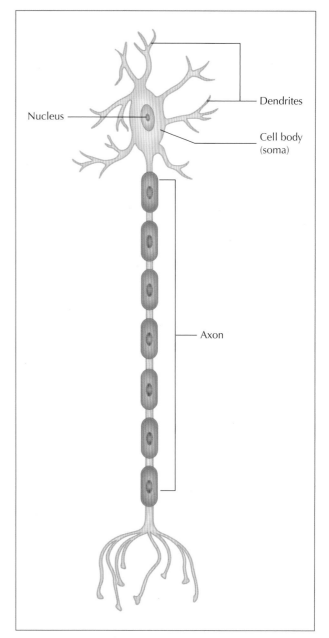

Figure 1.3: *A typical neuron with its associated cell body, axon, and dendrites (with dendritic spines).*

- *Multipolar*
- *Bipolar*
- *Unipolar*
- *Pseudo unipolar*

The majority of all neurons within the nervous system are *multipolar* and contain one axon and many dendrites; this type of neuron will be the focus of this text. *Bipolar neurons* are rare and found within the retina of the eye, while *unipolar neurons* are sensory neurons, found within

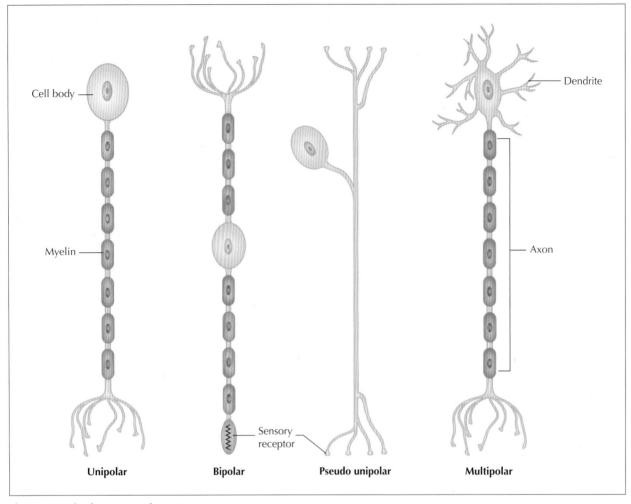

Figure 1.4: *The four types of neuron.*

the cell bodies of the spinal and cranial nerve ganglia (a collection of sensory neurons), and have only one structure projecting from the cell body. *Pseudo unipolar neurons* mainly constitute the sensory neurons and share similar characteristics with bipolar and unipolar neurons. They have a single structure from the cell body (as in the case of unipolar neurons), which branches into two separate structures: one extension that is connected to the dendrites, which inherently receive information, and another that transmits information to the spinal cord.

Within the nervous system, we generally say that there are three different classifications of neuron, dictated by their specific function:

1. Sensory neurons
2. Motor neurons
3. Interneurons

Sensory Neurons

Sensory neurons, which are also referred to as *afferent neurons*, simply transmit information from the sensory signals. This information typically derives from the physical inputs of sound, touch, heat, cold, pain, and light, vibration, proprioception, as well as from the chemical signals associated with smell and taste, originating from receptors in the body; the sensory neurons relay these signals *to* the CNS. Most sensory neurons are pseudo unipolar in nature, which means that they have only one axon and a structure that splits into two separate branches.

Motor Neurons

Motor neurons (or *motoneurons*), also referred to as *efferent neurons*, have the opposite function of sensory neurons: they transmit information *from* the CNS to the effectors of the body, such as the glands and skeletal muscles.

Motor neurons within the spinal cord are part of the CNS and they connect to the skeletal and smooth muscles, glands, and internal organs. There are two types of motor neuron: the ones that actually travel from the spinal cord directly to the muscles are known as *lower motor neurons*, and those that travel to and from the spinal cord toward the brain are known as *upper motor neurons*. Typically, motor neurons are multipolar, meaning that they have one axon with many attached dendrites.

Interneurons

Interneurons, also called *association neurons*, are only found in the CNS (brain or spinal cord) and are not found within the PNS. For example, a spinal interneuron located within the gray matter of the spinal cord will relay signals between an incoming afferent sensory neuron and an outgoing efferent motor neuron, a process called *sensory-motor integration*. These neurons connect or link the sensory and motor neurons together; they actually bridge the gap, because they are located between two neurons (one incoming neuron and one outgoing neuron). Interneurons are multipolar and also have the ability to communicate with other interneurons.

Neurons Within the Brain

The neurons that are actually located within the brain are very difficult to distinguish as compared to other neurons. For example, neurons located within the peripheral or central nervous system of the spinal cord can be easily recognized, as their type can identified on the basis of their function, which is a relatively straightforward process. The brain, however, has potentially hundreds of different types of neuron, and separating these in order to ascertain if they are sensory or motor neurons is near impossible. Researchers are still trying to work this out—a process that will no doubt take a very long time.

Interesting Facts about Neurons

Neurons are some of the longest-living cells within your body and will basically live as long as you do. They are irreplaceable, unlike some other cells in the body (e.g., skin cells), which have the ability to regenerate time and time again; they also have insatiable appetites, like a teenager who is growing and continually raiding the fridge to eat all the food. Neurons are essentially all based on the same structure and have a high metabolic rate, so they need an abundance of oxygen and glucose (calories) to maintain their function.

Nerves

Basically speaking, a *nerve* is the primary structure and only found within the PNS. Each nerve is composed of nerve bundles called *fascicles*, which contain hundreds of individual nerve fibers known as *neurons*.

A *peripheral nerve* contains the following structures (Figure 1.5):

- Axon
- Epineurium
- Endoneurium
- Endoneurial fluid
- Perineurium
- Fascicles
- Glycocalyx
- Myelin sheath

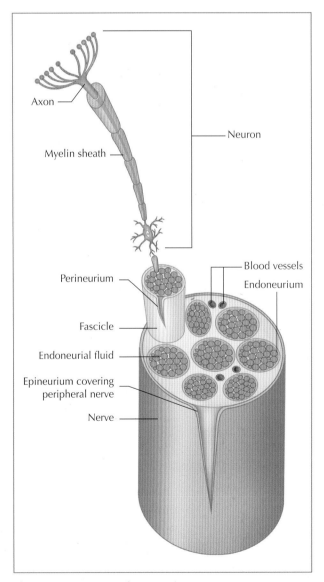

Figure 1.5: *Structure of a nerve.*

Axon

An *axon* is a long slender projection (think of a long cable) of a nerve cell or neuron, and is commonly known as the *nerve fiber*. The axon is many times thinner than a human hair and its function is to relay messages (electrical impulses called *action potentials*) away from the neurons cell body to other neurons, glands, and muscles. A neuron tends to have one axon but can interconnect with other neurons; some axons can travel a long way, for example from the spinal cord all the way down to the foot, although some can be only 0.04″ (1mm) in length. Axons make contact with other neurons as well as with muscle and gland cells, and these junction points are called *synapses*; this is a contact link between an axon terminal on one side and the dendrite or cell body on the other.

Axons also form side branches called *axon collaterals*; these extra projections (roots of a tree) are used to send signals to other neurons. The collaterals also split into what are referred to as *terminal branches*, each having a synaptic terminal on the tip. Longer axons in the peripheral nervous system tend to have a fatty insulating layer around them called *myelin* (which makes the brain matter white); this white fatty substance is produced by a Schwann cell (a type of glial cell), to form a sheath called a *myelin sheath*, as shown in Figure 1.6. This unique myelin sheath helps to speed up the signals, especially over longer distances.

Epineurium

The *epineurium* is simply the structure that forms the outermost covering of a peripheral nerve; it is like the outer "skin" of the spinal nerve and is made up of a layer of dense connective tissue.

Endoneurium

The *endoneurium* is the layer surrounding the actual axons and is formed by a layer of connective tissue.

Endoneurial Fluid

The *endoneurial fluid* is similar in one respect to the cerebrospinal fluid (CSF) of the CNS; however, this fluid is made up of a low protein liquid and is related in this instance to the PNS.

Perineurium

The *perineurium* is another covering of connective tissue, and this particular sheath covers the nerve fascicles.

Fascicles

Fascicles are simply a small bundle of nerve fibers that are encased within the protective sheath of the perineurium.

Glycocalyx

Glycocalyx is basically the "slime layer" that surrounds all of the cell membranes (think about when you pick up a fish, and you can feel all the slime on the outside); it is made up of a *glycoprotein* (carbohydrate chains attached to protein chains) and *glycolipid* (carbohydrate chains attached to fat chains) layer. Glycocalyx basically protects from certain invading types of bacterium and also controls the regulation of healthy cells against diseased or invading cells.

Myelin Sheath

The *myelin sheath* acts as an insulation layer that is wrapped around the axon and protects the axon. The sheath also increases the conduction (speed) of the electrical signals traveling through the axon; without this sheath, it is thought that the signals from the

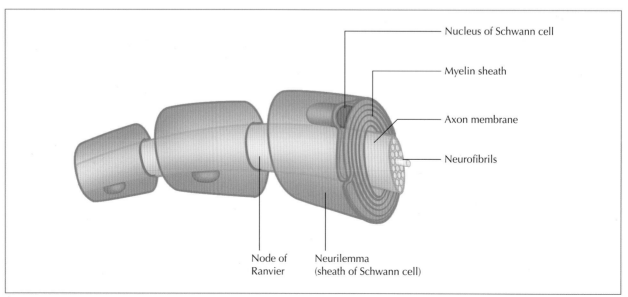

Figure 1.6: *An axon with a myelin sheath and Schwann cells.*

brain might not actually reach the muscles of the lower limb.

If you look at Figure 1.7, you can see how a single neuron is located within the nerve structure. The cell body is the "headquarters" of the neuron and its life-support system; it contains the nucleus, mitochondria, and genetic information in the form of DNA. You can see the dendrites (tree-like structures) sticking out from the cell body, which are responsible for receiving signals *from* other neurons and sensory cells. The axon transmits signals *away* from the cell body to other neurons, as I mentioned earlier, and can vary in length from very short (0.04″/1mm) to very long (40″/1m, or more).

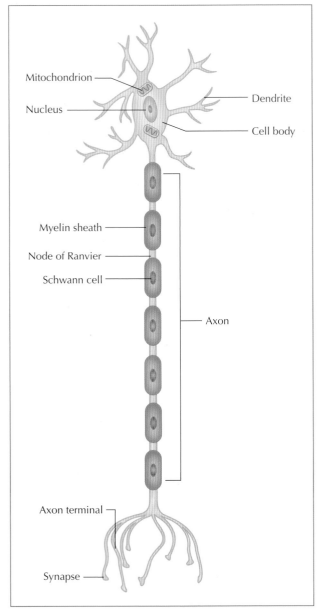

Figure 1.7: *A neuron, with its axon, dendrites, and cell body.*

Glial Cells

Around the neurons there are other cells called *glial cells* (from the Greek word 'glia' meaning 'glue'), which are designed to basically protect the neurons (like a bodyguard); they can be viewed as the "scaffolding" or the "glue" that holds and supports the neuron structure, as shown in Figure 1.8(a). They also provide nutrition and insulation as well as helping with the transmission of signals. Glial cells found within the PNS consist of only of two types: *satellite cells*, as shown in Figure 1.8(b), which surround the cell body of the neuron, and *Schwann cells*, which assist in the production of the myelin sheath and also provide insulation.

Glial cells are found in abundance within the CNS, and it has been considered that 50% of the mass of your brain is made up of these cells, outnumbering neurons by a ratio of approximately 10:1. For example, there are glial cells called *astrocytes* (star shaped); these link the neurons within the CNS to the blood capillaries, allowing an exchange of materials, as shown in Figure 1.9. The astrocytes also form the blood-brain barrier, which prevents harmful substances from entering the brain. There are also glial cells called *microglial cells*; these cells are protective in nature and defend against invading microorganisms within the brain and spinal cord. Basically, without the actions of the glial cells, neurons would cease to function, and when glial cells start to malfunction, then disaster occurs; for example, brain tumors are typically caused by a mutation of the glial cells.

The difference between a neuron and a glial cell is that a neuron contains an axon and dendrites and produces action potentials, whereas a glial cell does not have this capability, as its role is to provide the support mechanism and allow correct functioning (housekeeping) of the neurons to which they are directly attached.

There are many other types of glial cell located within the CNS, but since it is not within the scope of this book to pursue discussions about the CNS, I will leave it there.

Physiology of Nerve Conduction

The nervous system, I believe, is very much taken for granted—we just expect it to work. For example, you are currently reading this book (and hopefully you are liking the content) and visually your eyes are taking in what you are looking at on the page; we can call this the *sensory input*, taken in through your eyes. Then, once you have read the

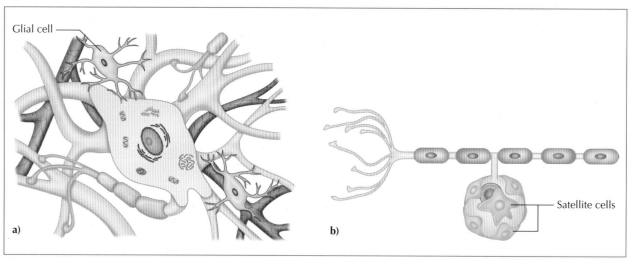

Figure 1.8: *(a) Example of a glial cell within the PNS. (b) A satellite cell.*

words on this page, the brain will decide (integration) what to do next; hopefully, the motor system will communicate with your fingers to turn to the next page.

Before you carry on reading, just pause for a moment and think about this action of being actually able to read the text, even though it is considered to be a simple task. What I want you to do now is to focus on your breathing, as that is part of your life-support system; without it we would simply die … not a nice thought, is it? Ask yourself the following questions … What is your body temperature? … Do you feel warm enough or are you a bit cold? … Is the seat you are sitting on making you feel comfortable, or do you want to stand up because you have been sitting for a few hours? Now stop and listen quietly to the sounds in the background; I am personally writing this text while listening to the birds in my garden, and now I am watching a squirrel scuttle past my window looking for nuts. All those things, plus a million more processes, are happening right here, right now, and most of them are

out of your control. Everything I have mentioned above is governed mainly by the nervous system—truly amazing, wouldn't you agree?

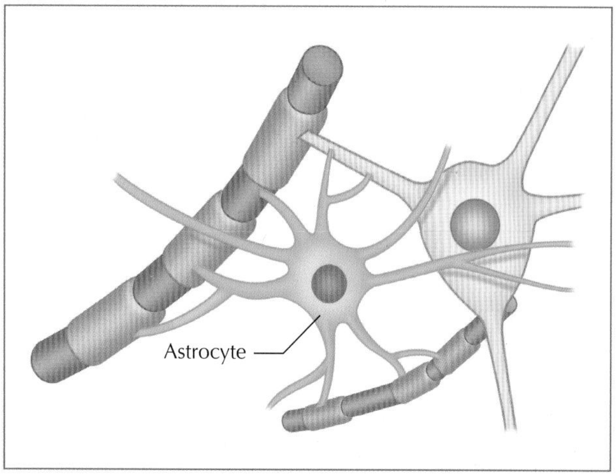

If our nervous system is operating normally, then, like everything in the workplace, it is all about good communication; it is similar to having a one-to-one discussion with your boss. With regard to the nervous system of the human body, communication is carried out between neurons, and there are over 100 trillion neural connections within the average brain. For communication to happen, there needs to be a signal sent (as well as the ability to receive it) to initiate the process. For example, the CNS sends a signal and the PNS will respond by continually sending the signal along the axon (train track) of the nerve fiber (neuron); this is typically performed by alpha motor neurons (large, multipolar lower motor neurons of the brainstem and spinal cord that innervate skeletal muscle fibers), and the electrical signal (train) can travel at speeds of up to approximately 270mph (431km/h)—pretty fast, agreed?

Before we get to the next stage, I just wanted to recap what I have covered so far, by means of an example of what is actually happening if, say, a spider walked across your leg. The sensory neurons within the skin on your leg would detect the motion of the spider, as would your visual senses located within your eyes (CN I, III, IV, VI). Naturally, the sensory signals from the skin of your leg will be transmitted via the axon, which is covered with a myelin sheath (which speeds up the signals), through the sensory afferent nerves, to the central nervous system of the spinal cord. When the information reaches the spinal cord, it will connect through many of the multipolar interneurons, some of which might automatically send signals down the

Figure 1.9: *Example of an astrocyte glial cell with the CNS.*

multipolar efferent lower motor neurons to send a signal to the quadriceps muscles to contract and to kick the leg, so that the spider falls off (spinal cord reflex). However, the information is also sent to the brain, via multipolar upper motor neurons, to recognize that a spider has contacted your skin. The brain will interpret those messages and then decide what to do next—which could be to simply scream or kick the leg—or the signals could come back and tell the person to relax and calm down and to slowly remove the spider from the leg. It sounds easy enough, but how does this process actually work?

Although each neuron has the capability of sending only one signal at a time with the same strength and speed, it is, however, able to change the frequency (number) of the signals; those impulses are known collectively as the *action potential* and will be discussed shortly.

So how does the electrical signal (voltage) travel along the axon (current)? I remember watching a video once, where the tutor described neurons to be like a bag of batteries, with each one having a *potential* to do something; for a simple task to be completed, a source of power is required and this is *electricity*. Each of these individual batteries has a positive and a negative side, and the potential to release energy; the same principle applies to the millions of individual neurons. The battery does not work, however, if it is not connected to anything or if it is flat (like with a flat battery in your car, the engine will not turn over). But, as soon as you connect the power supply to something, then it will work—for example, a torch will light or a child's toy will operate. Basically, each neuron in the body is like a single battery with a separate charge, and it will need something like an *event* to trigger and bring those charges together.

Within each neuron, the outer covering along the axon is called the *cell membrane*, and this structure separates the positive and negative charges. In a resting state, nothing really happens and the neuron is referred to as a *resting neuron*, as shown in Figure 1.10; there are no signals traveling down the axon, which is known as the *resting membrane potential* (RMP) and is normally measured to be around –70mv. The cells located within the neuron are relatively negatively charged compared with the outside of the membrane, where the cells are more positively charged, as shown in Figure 1.10.

Outside the neuron, the space is called *extracellular*, whereas inside the neuron it is known as *intracellular*. There are lots of ions present within these spaces, and in particular there is an abundance of sodium ions (NA^+), which are positively charged (+); generally speaking, there are more of these located outside the cell membrane than inside the cell. Inside the membrane of the neuron, there are more potassium ions (K^+) and these ions are also positively charged; however, the potassium ions are linked with larger and negatively charged (–) proteins. Overall, there are more sodium ions outside the cell membrane than there are potassium ions inside (linked with the larger negative proteins). This effect causes the inside of the cell to become more negatively charged, a state referred to as *polarized*.

Sodium–Potassium Pumps and Voltage-gated Potassium (K^+) Channels

All electrical events taking place within the neurons are controlled simply by the movement of ions. To allow this to happen we need some assistance, and there are unique pumps and channels that help in the process. These pumps are called *sodium–potassium pumps*, as shown in

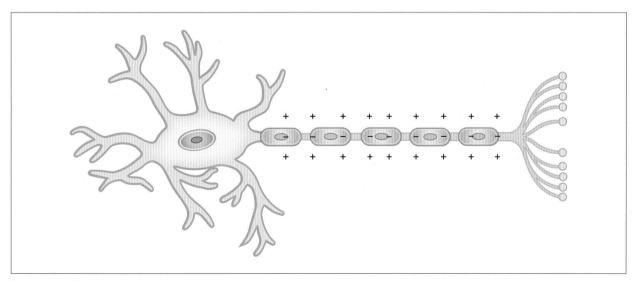

Figure 1.10: *Resting neuron.*

Figure 1.11(a), and are located in the cell membrane of the neuron; there are lots of these unique pumps located all the way along the axon. However, to assist the sodium–potassium pumps there are also other types of *entry* and *exit* channels, which penetrate the cell membrane and allow the passage of ions. One of these passages is called a *voltage-gated channel*, as shown in Figure 1.11(b), and these "flood gates" will open and close according to electrical changes in the cell membrane.

Action Potential

Let's look at an example of how the sodium–potassium pumps work. Roughly speaking, for every two potassium ions pumped into the cell (by the sodium–potassium pump), there will be three sodium ions pumped out, which will alter the electrical gradient. As mentioned earlier, this passage of ions will be the main function of all the electrical events within each neuron. For a substantial change in the electrical activity within the neuron, we need something called an *action potential*, and this will only happen when the neuron becomes *depolarized* (less negatively charged). There will need to be something major for this process of depolarization to happen, for example, touching something very hot, or if a spider walks across your leg. In such cases, the sodium ions quickly rush in through the pumps and also pass through the voltage-gated potassium (K^+) channels. Once the threshold of −55mv has been exceeded, the positive charge state continues to rapidly increase within the cell membrane (+40mv); this in turn causes an action potential (Figure 1.12) and sets up a chain reaction that continues all the way down the axon.

Once depolarization has occurred, then the next stage in this process is *repolarization*, as shown in Figure 1.13. This is where the potassium ions now escape through the voltage-gated potassium (K^+) channels, thus making the cell membrane more negatively charged and bringing back a balance to the electrical charge state. The process of depolarization and repolarization takes place during what is called the *refractory period*, and this process makes sure that each action potential is a unique event, also known as the *all or nothing event*.

If only a weak stimulus is present, however, then *action potentials* are less frequently activated. For example, when your brain says to your fingers to pick up a coin or a pen from your desk, it will stimulate a lower frequency than that for lifting up a heavy box from the ground or for squeezing someone's hand firmly; in the latter case, the stimulus is greater in order to alert more muscles to contract harder to lift the box or to squeeze the hand. The speed of signal conduction has been shown to increase substantially depending on the diameter of the axon: a larger diameter axon will allow greater speed of the signals traveling along it, so that action potentials will be allowed to happen much quicker.

Myelin Sheath and the Nodes of Ranvier

Within the PNS there is an amazing structure called the *myelin sheath*, which was briefly discussed earlier. The sheath speeds up the conduction of the signals traveling through the axon, by almost allowing the signals to "leap"

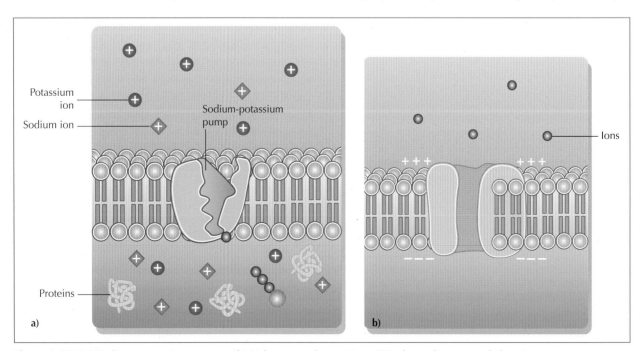

Figure 1.11: *(a) Sodium–potassium pumps. (b) Voltage-gated potassium (K^+) channels open and close in response to changes in membrane potential.*

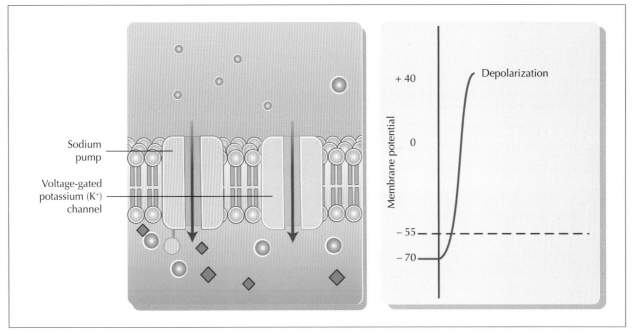

Sodium pump

Voltage-gated potassium (K⁺) channel

Figure 1.12: *Action potential causing depolarization.*

from one gap within the sheath to the next, as shown in Figure 1.14. These naturally formed gaps between the myelin sheath are known as the *nodes of Ranvier*, named after the French anatomist Louis-Antoine Ranvier; the leaping effect between the nodes is called *saltatory conduction* (from the Latin *saltare* meaning "to leap"

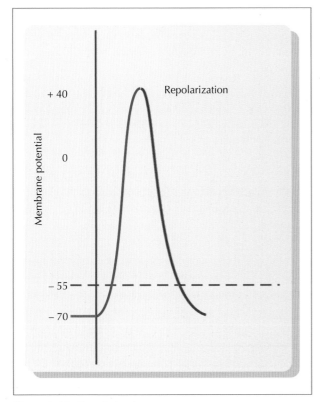

Figure 1.13: *Repolarization.*

or "to jump"). The concept of gaps along the myelin means that an axon has an access point to the outside cellular structure, whereby it can now utilize extra action potentials by adding in more voltage-gated potassium (K⁺) channels to allow the passage of the ions across these gaps. This process is basically a *signal booster*, and especially useful if the axon is very long; without the booster, the signal would be very weak by the time it got to the end of its lengthy journey.

Synapses

The ongoing mechanism by which neurons communicate with each other is similar, in my view, to what happens when we use our cell phones. If we text someone, or make a phone call to a friend (a process that is becoming less frequent), then it is a discussion between two people only; however, it is also possible to have a group discussion (by text or phone) with many people all at the same time. This technological capability is shared by the physiological structures called *synapses*; it is basically how neurons *talk* to each other! Sir Charles Scott Sherrington, a British neurophysiologist, first introduced the concept of synapses in 1897.

Neurotransmitters

So how do the synapses actually talk to each other? When two neurons come together, or when one neuron is in contact with a target cell (a muscle or gland), it is initially like saying that there is a break in the line of communication (a break in the train track). For an

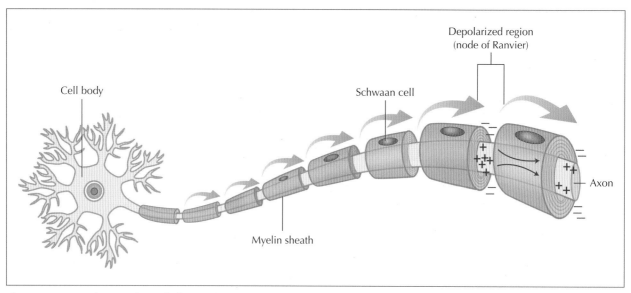

Figure 1.14: *Conduction through the myelin sheath, and the nodes of Ranvier.*

electrical signal to continue its journey and travel along the axon, it will need the ability to bridge the space naturally formed by the two neurons (the *synaptic cleft*). For this process to happen, the electrical signal in the majority of cases will need to be converted to a *chemical signal*, and this is the role of the *neurotransmitter*. Neurotransmitters have the ability to convert electrical signals to chemical signals, and then back again to electrical signals.

There are billions of neurons located within the nervous system and they will all need the actions of neurotransmitters in order to maintain all-round communication. Once this process of conversion has taken place, the signal can continue its journey and pass through the gap, which in this case is referred to as the *synapse* (Figure 1.15); this small space is actually considered to be around a millionth of an inch wide, or a thousand times thinner than a piece of paper! Can you imagine?

At the synapse, the sending cell, known as the *pre-synaptic cell*, transmits a signal to the receiving cell, known as the *post-synaptic cell*; this signal can be to either stimulate or inhibit the target neurons. More often than not, the transmission at the synapse is chemical based, but it can be electrical if a faster message is required, although less common. In terms of communication at the synapse, the chemical synapses are more in control, greater in number, slower to act, and generally more precise and more selective (they choose where to send the messages) than the electrical synapses (in cardiac muscle, for example, electrical signals are required).

As mentioned above, chemical transmission involves the neurotransmitters, and these messengers carry information from the pre-synaptic neuron to the post-synaptic neuron. A single axon can have many branches that connect to lots of post-synaptic neurons, and many thousands of inputs can be received all at the same time. Within the terminal of the axon of the pre-synaptic neuron are structures called *synaptic vesicle sacs*, which are filled with thousands of molecules from the neurotransmitter. The space formed between the end of the pre-synaptic neuron and the membrane of the post-synaptic neuron is known as the *synaptic cleft*, as shown in Figure 1.16. Just to clarify, this space is where the neurotransmitters pass through from the axon terminals (pre-synaptic) and are received at the receptor region of the receiving cell (post-synaptic). The two neurons never actually contact each other, as they are separated by the synaptic cleft.

The question is, how does the electrical signal change to a chemical signal across the synaptic cleft? Basically, when the action potentials (signals) are being sent along the axon, they activate the sodium–potassium pumps and voltage-gated channels, releasing sodium and potassium, before eventually reaching the axon terminals of the pre-synaptic neuron. This is where it starts to get interesting, because the voltage-gated *calcium* (Ca^{2+}) channels within the cell membrane now become activated (Figure 1.17); the positively charged calcium (Ca^{2+}) ions, which are higher in concentration outside the neuron, are allowed to pass directly through the channel and into the cell.

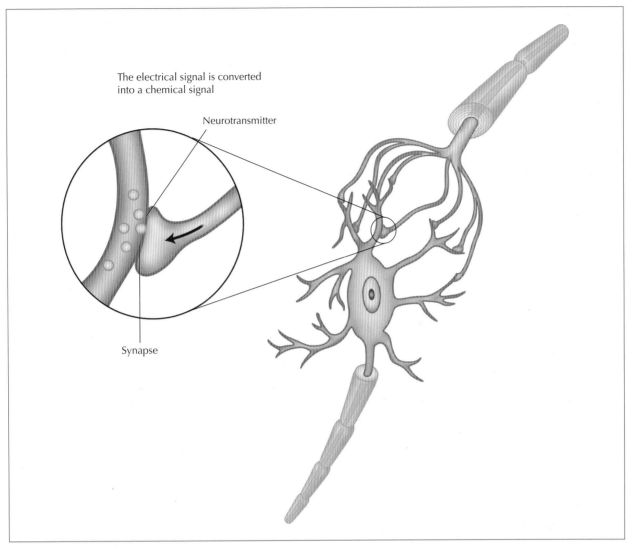

The electrical signal is converted into a chemical signal

Neurotransmitter

Synapse

Figure 1.15: *Synapse between neurons.*

The increased calcium now allows the synaptic vesicles to fuse with the axon terminal membrane. Subsequently, molecules of the neurotransmitter are released within the synaptic cleft and now cross the gap and bind to the post-synaptic neuron; this is the receiving cell, which is either the dendrite or the cell body, as shown in Figure 1.18.

Once the neurotransmitter has bonded to the receiving cell, the chemical signal will need to be converted back to an electrical signal in order to continue its journey as an action potential. However, at this stage, there are other choices, as it all basically depends on which particular neurotransmitter binds to which receptor: they can either cause the receiving neuron to get *excited* or *inhibited* (switch on or switch off—like a light), and this is dependent on the opening or closing of the ion channels. If an action potential signal is required (switch on), then

the signal to the target cell will be an excitatory (positive) one; the positive charge within the cell membrane of the post-synaptic neuron is increased, thus setting up the continuation of the electrical signal to the next neuron. On the other hand, if the opposite effect is required (switch off), the neurotransmitter is capable of changing its effect and making the cell membrane more negatively charged; this will cause an inhibitory (negative) signal, which basically means that the next neuron is not excited and the messages will stop there. Once neurotransmitters have delivered their messages, most of them are reabsorbed.

In simple terms, a *neurotransmitter* can be defined as a chemical released by the pre-synaptic neuron that will either excite or inhibit the post-synaptic neuron; this effect on the post-synaptic neuron happens in less than a millisecond. There are considered to be

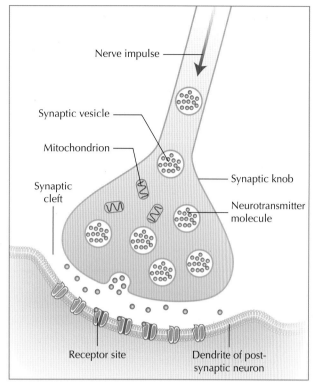

Figure 1.16: *Synapse and the synaptic cleft (space).*

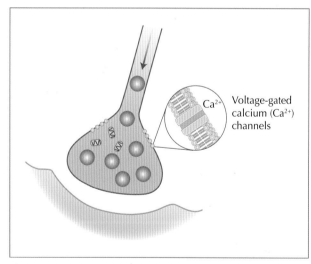

Figure 1.17: *Voltage-gated calcium (Ca²⁺) channels at the synapse.*

over one hundred different types of neurotransmitter within our bodies, serving many different functions: they can excite us or do the opposite and calm us down, they can make us sleepy, and they can control the function of the vital organs, as well as performing a multitude of other tasks. Four examples of types of neurotransmitter are:

- *Serotonin*, which basically causes an inhibitory effect and controls things like appetite, mood, and sleep.

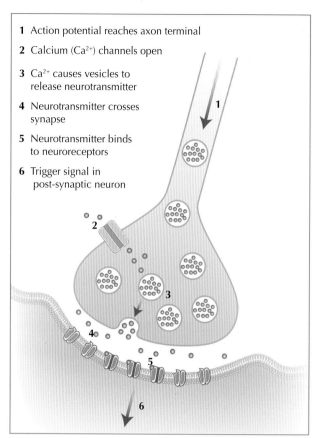

1. Action potential reaches axon terminal
2. Calcium (Ca²⁺) channels open
3. Ca²⁺ causes vesicles to release neurotransmitter
4. Neurotransmitter crosses synapse
5. Neurotransmitter binds to neuroreceptors
6. Trigger signal in post-synaptic neuron

Figure 1.18: *Physiology of neurotransmitters crossing the synaptic cleft and passing to the receiving cell (post-synaptic neuron).*

- *Dopamine*, which, when released, will make you feel amazing and increase your attention span.
- *Norepinephrine*, which relates to the fight or flight response, and increases respiration and heart rate.
- *Acetylcholine* (ACh), which is one of the main neurotransmitters and plays a major role in transmitting information within the PNS. ACh is released by motor neurons, as well as by pre-ganglionic sympathetic and parasympathetic neurons (see Chapter 2).

Neural Supercomputer

An interesting fact about synapses is that, because there are approximately 100 billion neurons within the brain and each neuron has between 1,000 and 10,000 synapses, there are a total of around 100–1,000 trillion synapses, each one of which is like a minicomputer, capable of changing and adapting, depending on the individual firing of the neurons!

2

Peripheral Nervous System

I t is amazing to think that we have 43 pairs of motor and sensory nerves which collectively make up the *peripheral nervous system* (PNS). This system, shown in Figure 2.1, links the all-important connections with the brain and spinal cord, known as the *central nervous system* (CNS); the main role of the PNS is to connect the CNS to the rest of the entire human body. Basically, all of the nerves and ganglia (a collection of sensory neurons) outside the brain and spinal cord are located within the PNS, and their role is to connect all the body structures—such as the organs, muscles, blood vessels, sensory organs, and glands—to the CNS.

The 43 pairs of motor and sensory nerves are split into:

- 31 pairs of spinal nerves
- 12 pairs of cranial nerves

Spinal nerves are further subdivided into:

- Cervical nerves—8 pairs (C1–C8)
- Thoracic nerves—12 pairs (T1–T12)
- Lumbar nerves—5 pairs (L1–L5)
- Sacral nerves—5 pairs (S1–S5)
- Coccygeal nerves—1 pair (Co1)

There are 12 pairs of cranial nerves, as listed in Table 2.1 and shown in Figure 2.2.

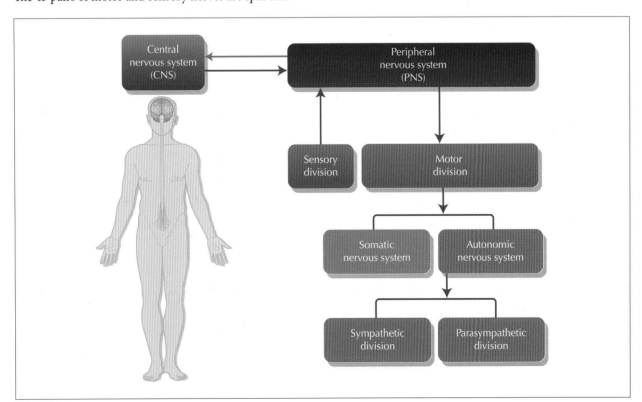

Figure 2.1: *The peripheral nervous system (PNS).*

Table 2.1: List of cranial nerves.

Number	Name of nerve	Nerve type	Function
I	Olfactory	Sensory	Smell
II	Optic	Sensory	Vision
III	Oculomotor	Motor	Most eye movement control
IV	Trochlear	Motor	Eye movement coordination (superior oblique muscle)
V	Trigeminal	Mixed	Face and mouth sensation, muscles of mastication control
VI	Abducens	Motor	Eye abduction (lateral rectus muscle)
VII	Facial	Mixed	Muscles of facial expression, lacrimal and salivary glands (taste)
VIII	Vestibulocochlear	Sensory	Hearing and balance
IX	Glossopharyngeal	Mixed	Gag reflex, sense of taste and serve the pharynx for swallowing
X	Vagus	Mixed	Gag reflex, control of heart, parasympathetic innervation of muscles of viscera
XI	Accessory	Motor	Shoulder shrugging and movement of neck
XII	Hypoglossal	Motor	Swallowing, speech, movement of tongue

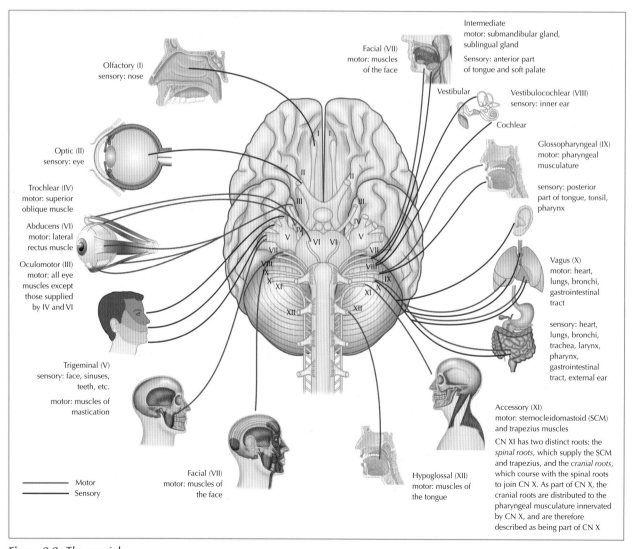

Figure 2.2: *The cranial nerves.*

■ Structure of the PNS—Sensory and Motor

The PNS is made up of two types of neuron—sensory and motor—which were briefly mentioned earlier. The text below, however, will discuss the function of these two neurons in a slightly different way and, more importantly, how they are interrelated, for example through the reflex arc.

Sensory (or Afferent) Neuron

Sensory neurons, also called *afferent neurons* (*afferent* means "toward the brain or spinal cord"), are responsible for detecting various sensations, for example heat, cold, and pain. The sensory neurons will then transmit these sensory messages directly *toward* the CNS via the PNS, and either the spinal cord or the brain will interpret these signals.

The sensory component of the PNS has many types of receptor that respond to sensory changes. Receptors that detect temperature changes are called *thermoreceptors*, and those that detect chemical changes are *chemoreceptors*. *Photoreceptors* detect changes in light, *mechanoreceptors* respond to changes in pressure, touch, and vibration, and lastly *nociceptors* react only to pain stimuli.

Motor (or Efferent) Neuron

Motor neurons, or *efferent neurons* (*efferent* means "away from the brain or spinal cord") are basically the opposite of the sensory neuron in one respect, because they will transmit messages directly *away* from the CNS. Their primary role is to stimulate effectors within the skin, organs, and of course the muscles, to either perform a function or a reflex.

Note that all of the 43 pairs of nerves (spinal and cranial) located within the PNS perform either sensory or motor functions, or a combination of both (mixed).

The Reflex Arc

Let me try to explain the messages that are sent from a sensory afferent neuron to a motor efferent neuron and how these two are linked together. It will be easier to discuss this process through the use of what is known as the *reflex arc*.

If you look at Figure 2.3, you will notice a stimulus from the sensory receptor of the foot (skin) as a result of standing on something sharp (pin); the signal is relayed via the sensory afferent neuron to the ganglia. The ganglia then send these messages directly to the dorsal part of the spinal cord (CNS). Once these messages have been processed, there is a natural link (interneuron) that connects to the motor efferent neuron (ventral part of the spinal cord), and this subsequently carries the response and is relayed to the effector; in this case, the muscles are instructed to contract, so that the foot can be lifted off the sharp object.

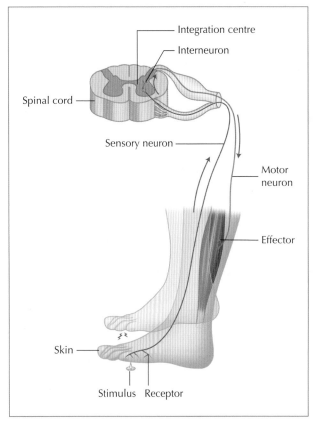

Figure 2.3: *Reflex arc.*

The ganglia messages (reflexes) are designed to be quick thinking and demand an automatic response, because they have your health in mind and are maintaining your body's self-preservation. They are acting as your personal bodyguard, and, basically, their simple primary role is to protect you from harm. These super quick reflexes are initiated and subsequently processed, all of which happens even before the pain is sensed at the brain level.

■ Divisions of the PNS

The PNS is subdivided into two separate systems: the voluntary division and the involuntary division.

The *voluntary division*, better known as the *somatic nervous system*, is consciously controlled, and its main responsibilities are to relay sensory and motor information between the outside environment and the CNS. This is mainly because of the ability of the somatic nerves to innervate the outer part of the body, such as the skeletal muscles and the skin. Naturally, any movement of the muscles or any voluntary output will utilize the somatic nervous system.

The *involuntary division*, better known as the *autonomic nervous system*, controls all of the vital body functions (heart rate, respiration, and digestion) as well as the innervation of the internal organs. The autonomic nervous system is outside of our conscious voluntary control, and all of these internal functions happen automatically.

■ The Autonomic Nervous System

The autonomic nervous system (ANS), as mentioned above, is an integral part of the PNS; its main action is to influence the function of the internal organs, and it does this by controlling the smooth muscle and cardiac muscle of the viscera and also the glands. The ANS is simply (in one respect) an automated process and has no conscious control. For example, when we place some food into our mouths and start to chew, we can consciously decide when to swallow; however, once that process is complete, the ANS kicks in to begin the digestion of the food in the stomach, where the bolus (food) is broken down automatically by the secretion of gastric juices. The nutrients are then passed and absorbed mainly through the small intestine, and eventually the waste (fecal matter) is discharged from the anus by a process called *defecation*.

No matter where you are or what you are doing, the ANS is continually working—there is no rest, no vacation, no time off, etc. The ANS is the body's fine-tuning system… try to relate this to an auto mechanic tuning your engine during a routine service, so that your automobile runs better and more efficiently!

Sympathetic and Parasympathetic Nervous Systems

The ANS is subdivided into another two systems: the sympathetic nervous system and the parasympathetic nervous system as shown in Figure 2.4. You have probably heard of the *fight or flight* mechanism; this unique mechanism is part of the *sympathetic nervous system* (SNS) (from Greek, meaning "feeling together")

and is responsible for exciting or stimulating the body. A second element, the lesser-known *rest and digest* mechanism, forms the other part of the ANS and is called the *parasympathetic nervous system* (PSNS) (from Greek, meaning "beside the sympathetic"). The PSNS is basically responsible for calming down the body and preserving energy for a later date.

Ganglia

The ANS and PSNS need two types of neuron to work correctly (see below), and these particular neurons are linked to structures called *ganglia*, which are groups of neurons that contain millions of synapses. The sympathetic ganglia are located a lot closer to the spinal cord than the parasympathetic ganglia; the latter are found much further away from the spine and even inside their effector organs.

The neurons that connect *from* the spinal cord of the CNS to the ganglia are called *pre-ganglionic neurons* (this includes both the sympathetic and parasympathetic division). All of these neurons are myelinated (i.e., have a myelin sheath), and they all use acetylcholine (ACh) as a neurotransmitter.

The neurons that connect *from* the ganglia to the effector cells are called *post-ganglionic neurons*. The SNS post-ganglionic axons are much longer than the shorter pre-ganglionic axons. The opposite is true in the case of the PSNS: the PSNS post-ganglionic neurons are a lot shorter than their longer pre-ganglionic neurons (see Figure 2.5).

Sympathetic Nervous System

The SNS originates from the thoracolumbar region of the body, which equates to the levels T1–T12 of the thoracic spine, and continues to approximately L2 of the lumbar spine; this is known as the *thoracolumbar outflow* (Figure 2.4).

Every single one of us has experienced a stress response at some point in our busy and stressful lives, and what we encounter is known as the *fight-or-flight response*. The problem with modern day society is that the scenario of our ancestors living in a prehistoric cave and having to either "fight" an animal (i.e., for survival or for food) or adopt the opposite strategy and perform "flight" (i.e., run away from the risk) is now a little unrealistic. However, the body does not know (or care) that you are living in a house or an apartment on the 10th floor and not living in

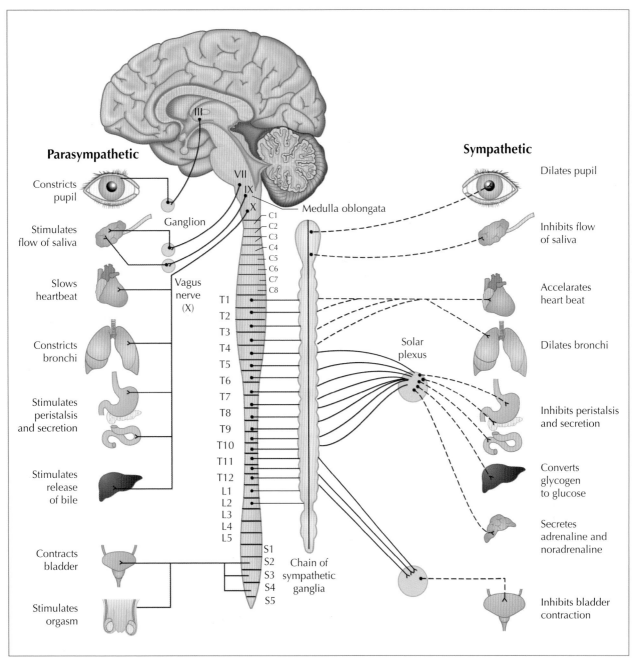

Figure 2.4: *Autonomic nervous system – sympathetic and parasympathetic.*

a cave anymore, and that you no longer fight with animals for food. To the body, a "stress" response reaction from the SNS will potentially be exactly the same, regardless of whether you are running from a lion on the Serengeti or simply in a "road rage" situation because the person in front of you nabbed your car parking spot at the grocery store.

The way I think about the sympathetic system is as follows. The "s" of "sympathetic" also stands for "stress," and when the sympathetic process is active, it will

typically allow the body to react to stressful situations. The SNS will achieve this by affecting the *whole* of the body's systems (i.e., not just one system, but many) in the following ways:

- Eyes—Dilates the pupils to enhance sight
- Mouth—Inhibits salivation
- Heart—Increases heart rate and blood pressure
- Lungs—Increases respiration rate through dilation (opening) of the bronchioles

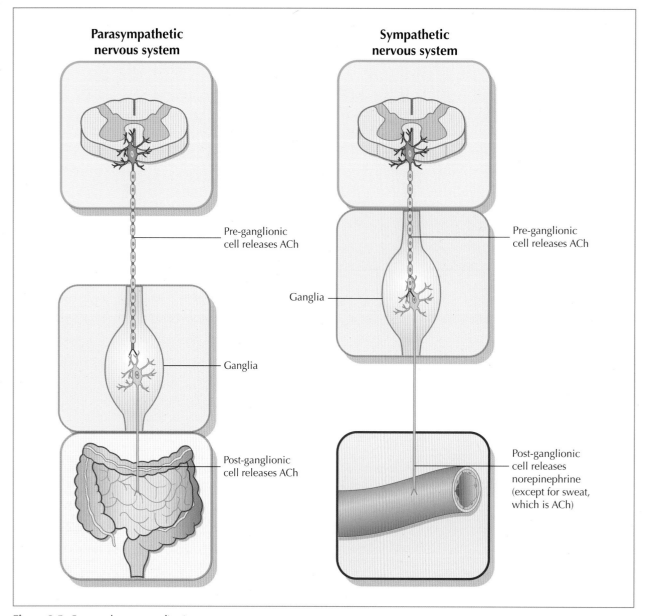

Figure 2.5: *Pre- and post-ganglionic neurons.*

- Stomach—Shuts down gastrointestinal function through vasoconstriction
- Liver—Releases glucose in preparation for physical response and inhibits the gallbladder
- Blood vessels—Diverts blood to the extremities through vasodilation
- Skin—Increases sweating
- Adrenal glands—Stimulates the release of norepinephrine and epinephrine
- Bladder—Relaxes the bladder
- Sexual glands—Promotes orgasm

There are four main stress response hormones and chemicals released from neurotransmitters and organs:

1. Acetylcholine
2. Norepinephrine
3. Epinephrine
4. Cortisol

Sympathetic Nervous System and Acetylcholine

When your body perceives a stress situation (fight or flight), the brain sends signals down the spinal cord. These messages exit through the intermediate lateral

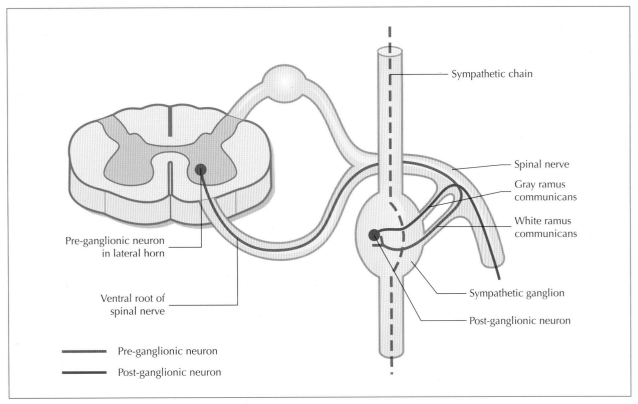

Figure 2.6: *Sympathetic nervous system ganglia (pre-ganglionic/post-ganglionic).*

gray horn located just within the thoracolumbar region of the sympathetic nervous system (T1–L2) of the spinal cord, which is where the cell bodies (which are called *pre-ganglionic*) of the sympathetic motor neurons are located, as shown in Figure 2.6. The information is sent along the ventral root (the same pathway as the peripheral/somatic nerve) to the ventral ramus, and passes through the tunnel called the *white ramus communicans (pl. white rami communicantes)* ("white" because it is myelinated), before entering the sympathetic ganglia, where hundreds of cell bodies are found.

You can see from Figure 2.7 that there are many other ganglia located above and below the one being described, and these are located along the sympathetic chain; these are known as *chain ganglia*, or *paravertebral ganglia*.

When the signals reach the synapses within the ganglia, the neurotransmitters release the chemical acetylcholine (ACh), of which there is an abundance within the CNS and PNS; ACh is the main chemical responsible for all of the communications between neurons. The signals are now sent to the *post-ganglionic neuron*, which exits through the tunnel called the *gray ramus communicans (pl. rami communicantes)* ("gray" because it is not

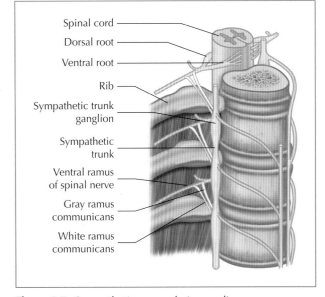

Figure 2.7: *Sympathetic nerve chain ganglia.*

myelinated) and follows the pathway of a peripheral spinal nerve. This passage of the post-ganglionic neuron subsequently causes a reaction in the effector cells; for example, it activates the smooth muscle tissue within the skin and makes our hairs "stand up straight" (*piloerection*) through the contraction of the arrector pili muscles; these

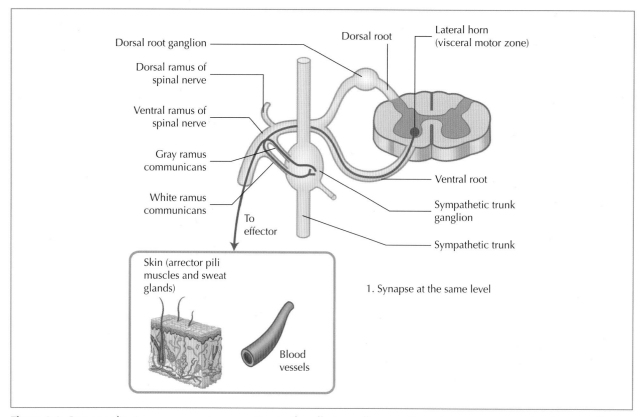

Figure 2.8: *Post-ganglionic neuron causing a reaction to the effector cells, e.g., pilomotor, vasomotor, and sudomotor fibers.*

are known as *pilomotor fibers* and contract all at once, as shown in Figure 2.8. Next, the stress response either causes a vasoconstriction of the blood vessels and reduces blood supply to certain parts of the body (gut), or causes the blood vessels to dilate, which will increase the flow of blood (skeletal muscles); these are called *vasomotor fibers*. The stress response also leads to another process—it controls our sweat glands and causes us to perspire; these are called *sudomotor fibers*. (There is an exception to the chemical release for the control of sweating: the post-ganglionic sympathetic fibers release the neurotransmitter acetylcholine (Ach) and not norepinehrine.)

Within the chain ganglia, the signals can be sent to other ganglia (this is simply to spread the signals—think of a group text) that are located above and below the original one that the signals entered beforehand, and also to synapses, before passing through the gray rami communicans (explained earlier), as shown in Figure 2.9.

Splanchnic Nerves

There is another way that the SNS sends messages to the effectors, such as the heart and the lungs of the thorax and even the head and neck, and this is through the generation of a nerve of its own, rather than the messages traveling in conjunction with a spinal nerve. After the signals have

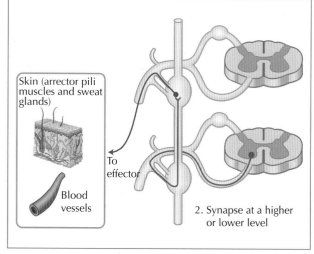

Figure 2.9: *Post-ganglionic neuron exiting the ganglia above the level of entry.*

passed through the white rami communicans and have synapsed through the cell bodies within the chain ganglia, the post-ganglionic fiber then passes out of the ganglia as a *splanchnic* nerve but they synapse later near the relevant organ. It does this directly from the chain ganglia without even exiting through the gray rami communicans; basically, this system has its own tunnel or tube that passes directly out of the original ganglia, as shown in Figure 2.10.

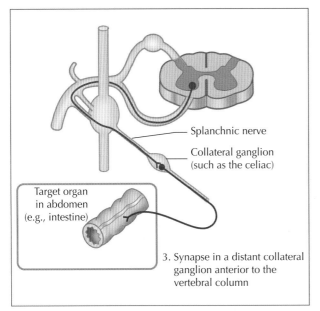

Splanchnic nerve

Collateral ganglion
(such as the celiac)

Target organ
in abdomen
(e.g., intestine)

3. Synapse in a distant collateral
ganglion anterior to the
vertebral column

Figure 2.10: *Signals traveling from the chain ganglia directly to the splanchnic ganglia.*

Pre-aortic Ganglia

Another concept I would like to discuss is that the signals can pass straight through the chain ganglia without actually synapsing at that level as explained earlier (the only ones that do not synapse are for the gut and adrenal gland). The neuron therefore maintains its status as a pre-ganglionic cell and exits through another separate tunnel, to continue its journey on to another type of ganglia called *pre-aortic, pre-vertebral* or *collateral ganglia* (Figure 2.11). From here, the signals leave as a post-ganglionic neuron via a splanchnic nerve, and these messages will directly affect the abdominal and pelvic visceral regions (*visceral* = "relating to the organs").

Norepinephrine

Norepinephrine, also called *noradrenalin*, is actually a hormone as well as a chemical neurotransmitter, and is released from post-ganglionic fibers to its effector cells. Its basic function is to prepare the body and the brain for action, especially during stressful times. The chemical

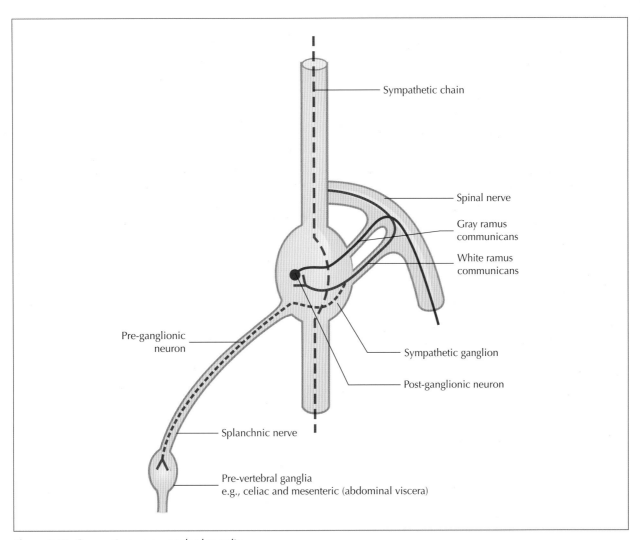

Sympathetic chain

Spinal nerve

Gray ramus
communicans

White ramus
communicans

Pre-ganglionic
neuron

Sympathetic ganglion

Post-ganglionic neuron

Splanchnic nerve

Pre-vertebral ganglia
e.g., celiac and mesenteric (abdominal viscera)

Figure 2.11: *Pre-aortic or pre-vertebral ganglia.*

is produced within the brain and also in some parts of the SNS. Generally speaking, norepinephrine is at its lowest level while we are sleeping; however, when we awaken it is then released and increases depending on the stress responses we perceive in our daily lives.

Norepinephrine mainly acts to increase the heart rate and blood pressure by causing the blood vessels to constrict (become narrower), as well as activating the release of glucose and increasing the flow of blood to the skeletal muscles and their contraction. (Noradrenalin is also a drug that can be injected into the blood stream to raise blood pressure, especially if you have something called *septic shock*, which can lead to organ failure.) The adrenal glands, located above the kidneys, can also release this chemical directly into the blood system if needed.

Epinephrine

Just to clarify: ACh is released from the *pre-ganglionic* neurons at the synapse, and norepinephrine is released from *post-ganglionic* neurons to the effector cells. The stress response also causes ACh to be released by the adrenal glands and this in turn causes the adrenal medulla to release two hormones, one called *norepinephrine* (a chemical neurotransmitter), which was discussed above, and another one called *epinephrine*, otherwise known as *adrenaline*.

An acute stressful response will cause an "adrenaline rush," which is very similar to the effect of norepinephrine, because epinephrine is also a neurotransmitter and a hormone, and will increase blood sugar levels as well as heart and respiration rates. The difference between the two is that norepinephrine can cause blood pressure to increase by narrowing the blood vessels, while epinephrine has a slightly greater effect on the heart; however, they are both involved extensively in the "fight or flight" response. It is interesting because epinephrine can have both a stimulating effect by increasing blood flow to certain parts of the body (such as the skeletal muscles) by causing the blood vessels to relax (which induces vasodilation and increases the flow of blood), and at the same time a relaxing effect by restricting and decreasing blood flow to other parts of the body where it is not needed (such as the stomach and small intestine) by causing the blood vessels to constrict (which induces vasoconstriction and decreases the flow of blood). In its synthetic form, epinephrine can be used for the treatment of, for example, anaphylaxis, an asthma attack or cardiac arrest.

Cortisol

Cortisol is a steroid hormone produced and released through the adrenal glands, and is the primary hormone (typically referred to as the *stress hormone*) released in response to stress. It causes blood sugar levels to increase and improves and regulates the metabolism of fats, proteins, and carbohydrates. Once a potential threat has passed, it is the function of cortisol to alert the body to replenish energy, which is normally achieved through the craving of sugary foods. Chronic and ongoing stress maintains higher than normal cortisol levels within your system; this can lead to many health-related conditions, such as weight gain, high blood pressure, headaches, muscle weakness, and thinning skin with poor healing capabilities. *Adrenal insufficiency* is basically a reduction in the hormone cortisol released from the adrenal glands. A condition called *Addison's disease* can manifest as a result of this insufficiency, with symptoms ranging from depression and weight and hair loss, to low blood pressure, low blood sugar, and muscle or joint pains.

Just for a moment, think about all of those bullet points listed earlier for the effects of the SNS on the body's systems and the way the stress chemicals are released. This is the way the body will react as a result of a stressful situation—do you not agree that it is truly amazing that the body is able to perform all of those functions, or possesses these natural instincts (as I sometimes say), and that these reactions occur *every* single time you are "stressed"?

The Stress Response—Good or Bad Thing?

An issue in today's society is that we commonly discuss stress in one of two ways—either *good stress* or *bad stress*. But, realistically, is there such a distinction? Because isn't stress just stress? I believe there is a major problem with stress and, in particular, with the way our body interprets it. Why? Because the problem is that a stress response is a natural process of the body; however, if we have continual and repeated stress triggers, especially on a daily basis, then I believe these phenomena will be detrimental to our overall well-being, and one might now call this *bad stress*.

A quick example: imagine yourself as a committed partner who works hard to provide for your family, as you have two young children, and you work in an office all day and have done for many years. Every day your boss gives you more work to deal with; you accept this extra work, and you are even happy to receive it because you want a promotion. However, in your heart you knew that you would struggle to finish the tasks on time. As a result of this, you end up spending longer in the office because of the extra workload, and when you arrive home, you still have to spend time on the PC because of work-related deadlines. I mentioned earlier that you were married with two children, and now you end up seeing less and less of them, so the relationship is suffering. The mortgage, car, and credit card debts and other loans are getting out of hand, so you borrow more money to pay off existing loans. Now you have just been told your mother is very ill and she needs urgent medical care; a care home has been suggested and naturally there is a high cost attached to that process. Imagine the above scenario… no doubt your adrenaline and cortisol, as well as other stress-related hormones, will be continually secreted from the adrenal glands. Sooner or later you might become *adrenal insufficient* and as a result be prescribed steroids and other medication to control your ever-increasing stress. This scenario is probably not the best way forward for maintaining overall good health and longevity; however, the situation I have discussed is not uncommon in today's stressful society.

One of the phrases I personally use to clarify the significance of stress is the following:

> *"Stress causes disease, and disease causes stress."*

Just to recap, the SNS system originates from the thoracic spine (T1–T12) and continues to approximately L2 of the lumbar spine—this is the thoracolumbar outflow. The SNS uses ACh at the pre-ganglionic neuron, and norepinephrine at the post-ganglionic neuron.

Parasympathetic Nervous System

As discussed earlier, the *parasympathetic nervous system* (PSNS) is typically referred to as the *rest and digest system*, because of its calming influences (from Greek, meaning "beside the sympathetic"). The system has also been known as the *cranial sacral system* or *cranio-sacral outflow*, because of its neurological origin from the cranium and the sacrum landmarks. Compared with the SNS, which is active in short bursts and generates immediate stress response signals, the PSNS is active most of the time. The PSNS has many continuous and necessary functions; for example, it promotes the digestion of food that you consume and then controls the way in which the body will excrete its waste (defecation), it maintains health by fighting off infections, and it facilitates cell reproduction.

The PSNS is responsible for the following reactions:

- Eyes—Constricts the pupils
- Mouth—Stimulates the flow of saliva
- Heart—Slows the heartbeat

- Lungs—Constricts the bronchioles
- Stomach—Stimulates peristalsis and secretion
- Liver—Inhibits the release of glucose and stimulates the gallbladder to release bile
- Bladder—Contracts the bladder, causes erection

The PSNS is made up of the following structures, forming the craniosacral outflow (Figure 2.12):

- CN III—Oculomotor nerve
- CN VII—Facial nerve
- CN IX—Glossopharyngeal nerve
- CN X—Vagus nerve
- Sacral division S2–S4

Note: Cranial nerves III, VII and IX are NOT parasympathetic nerves themselves but each of them

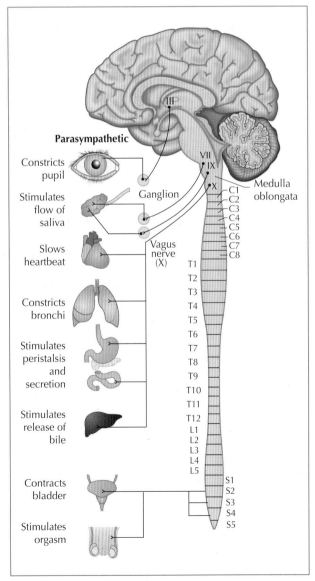

Figure 2.12: *Parasympathetic nervous system (PSNS).*

CARRY parasympathetic fibers from the three parasympathetic nuclei in the brain stem. The vagus nerve itself is pure parasympathetic but, of course, carries various other fibers.

Naturally, all of the cranial nerves are important; however, there is one in particular that needs mentioning and discussing, and that, as you have probably guessed, is the vagus nerve (CN X), as shown in Figure 2.13.

The *vagus nerve* is responsible for almost 90% of the information sent through the PSNS: it sends sensory messages to the brain, and transmits motor messages from the brain back to the body. The nerve is purely parasympathetic and carries sensory fibers: general visceral afferent and somatic sensory, and works automatically, without our conscious control, as shown in Figure 2.14. There are general visceral sensory (afferent) fibers that run adjacent to CN X and detect hunger, fullness, pain, and inflammation. However, they are not part of the autonomic nervous system (ANS), which is all motor.

Differences Between the SNS and the PSNS

One of the main differences between the SNS and the PSNS lies in the release of chemicals. I discussed earlier that the SNS releases the chemical *norepinephrine* at the post-ganglionic neurons to the effector cells; however, the PSNS releases *ACh* from the post-ganglionic neurons to the effector cells. The SNS and PSNS and the somatic nervous system are outlined in the flow chart in Figure 2.15.

Let's return to the example from earlier, in which you imagined yourself to be the man or woman who was stressed out every day when at work and struggling with your finances and home life. When you came home in the evening, you would no doubt want to relax, watch some TV, and eat some dinner. As you start to eat the food, the vagus nerve becomes active, sending signals (sensory) from the stomach to the brain to say that there is food present and that the stomach is filling up; the food is then broken down in the stomach, which is a natural

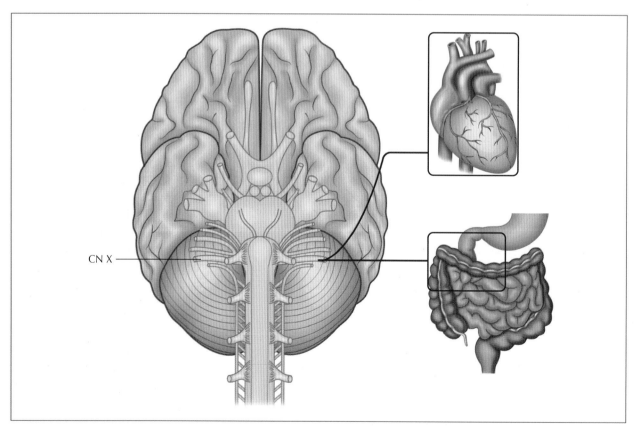

Figure 2.13: *CN X – Vagus nerve – controls the heart and digestive tract amongst other functions.*

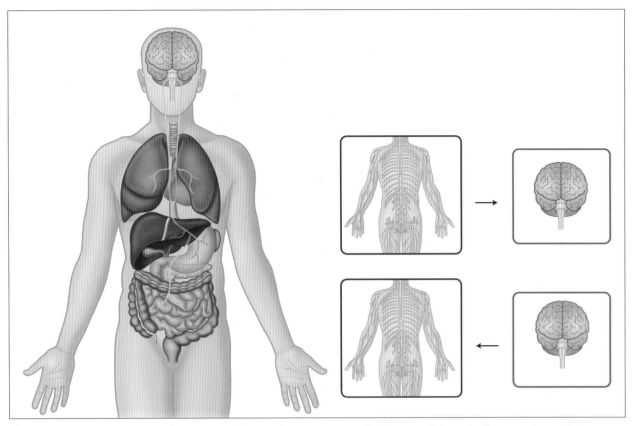

Figure 2.14: *Vagus nerve is purely parasympathetic and carries sensory fibers: general visceral afferent and somatic sensory.*

parasympathetic action. The vagus nerve also sends messages (motor) to other areas of the body—signals, for example, to transport glucose to areas of storage so that they can be used at a later date; to reduce heart and respiration rates; and to limit the amount of norepinephrine released by the SNS. The result—you now feel a lot more relaxed! The possible negative side of this, though, is that eating food to excess is some people's way of reducing their stress levels… we call it *comfort eating.*

The PSNS is the system that is in control and the dominant one in the relationship, as it is basically trying to limit the action of the SNS. Take, for example, the case of a caged wild animal: the metal cage is the PSNS and the wild animal inside is the SNS. Now and again, we have to let the animal out of the cage to run around and get rid of its stress; hopefully, once the stress has been released, the animal (sympathetic) will go back to its cage to rest. Wouldn't it be an amazing and rather simple existence if life was like that? However, we know for a fact that life is

complex and not that simple at all, and that a caged animal does not usually want to go back to its cage, as it likes to roam outside. And let's be honest, who would blame it, as every human has a unique story to tell and some stories are potentially more stressful than others.

Let's look at a simple example of how to influence the PSNS, and more importantly how to calm a caged animal. If you are feeling anxious or nervous about something, you will probably be aware of (and able to feel) your heart and respiration rate starting to increase. In such an event, try the following simple exercise. Many watches (Apple, Fitbit, etc.) can continuously measure your heart rate, so look at the heart reading on the watch while trying to consciously control your breathing. Start by slowly taking in a deep inhalation, hold the breath at the end for 1–2 seconds, then breathe out deeply. Repeat this process 5–10 times, during which you will notice your heart rate begin to lower. This action is down to the PSNS, which it performs automatically, even though you are controlling and focusing on your breathing technique.

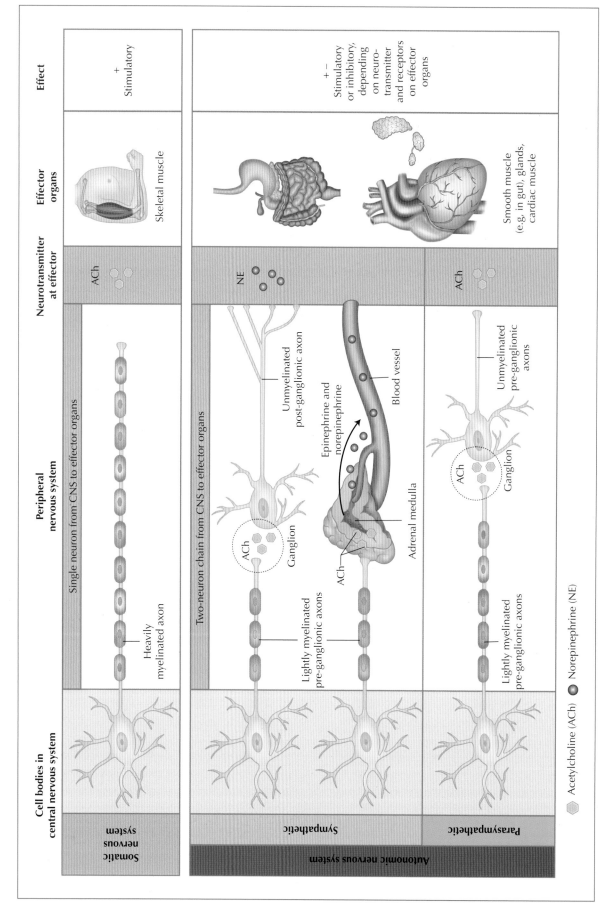

Figure 2.15: *Somatic, sympathetic, and parasympathetic flow chart.*

⬡ Acetylcholine (ACh)   ⬤ Norepinephrine (NE)

3

Anatomy and Function of the Cervical and Brachial Plexuses

In this chapter the focus will be on the two nerve plexuses that directly affect the neck and upper limb; known individually as the *cervical plexus* and *brachial plexus*. You will notice in the following text that the majority of the discussion will concentrate on the brachial plexus, as this book has been written mainly with the physical therapist in mind and because patients naturally tend to present with conditions typically located within the structure of this particular plexus. The cervical plexus is just as important, however, and will be discussed first but only relatively briefly.

■ Cervical Plexus

The cervical plexus (Figure 3.1) is a network of nerves, formed by the anterior primary rami of the four upper cervical nerves (C1–4). This plexus is located within the neck, deep to the sternocleidomastoid, and has both cutaneous and muscular branches.

The cervical plexus can simply be categorized into *muscular branches* and *sensory branches*.

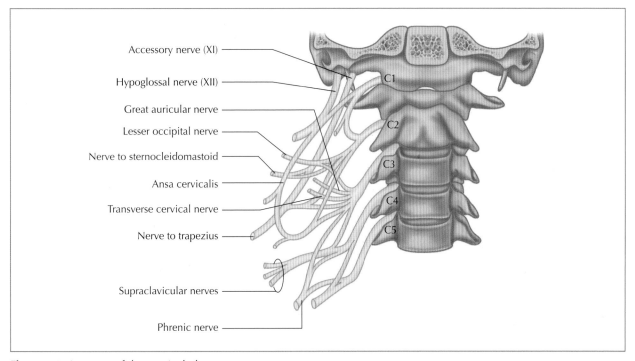

Accessory nerve (XI)
Hypoglossal nerve (XII)
Great auricular nerve
Lesser occipital nerve
Nerve to sternocleidomastoid
Ansa cervicalis
Transverse cervical nerve
Nerve to trapezius
Supraclavicular nerves
Phrenic nerve

C1
C2
C3
C4
C5

Figure 3.1: *Anatomy of the cervical plexus.*

Muscular Branches

The C1 spinal nerve innervates the geniohyoid muscle, which assists in expanding the airway by moving the hyoid bone upward and anteriorly. C1 also innervates the thyrohyoid muscle and this assists in depressing the hyoid bone, resulting in elevation of the larynx.

C1–3 form the "goose neck," medically termed the *ansa cervicalis*, and gives off four muscular branches that supply the muscles collectively known as the *infrahyoids*; these muscles assist in swallowing and speech and do this by depressing the hyoid bone. The infrahyoids consist of:

1. Sternothyroid
2. Sternohyoid
3. Omohyoid (superior belly)
4. Omohyoid (inferior belly)
5. Thyrohyoid

C3–5 Phrenic Nerve
The most notable nerve that constitutes part of the muscular branch is the *phrenic nerve*, which supplies the diaphragm and originates from C3, C4, and C5. A little saying to remember this is: "C3, 4, 5, keep the diaphragm alive."

Traveling from its origin in the cervical region of C3–5, the phrenic nerve passes over the anterior fibers of the scalenes, penetrates the thorax cavity, and descends to the base of the lung, before finally reaching the diaphragm (Figure 3.2).

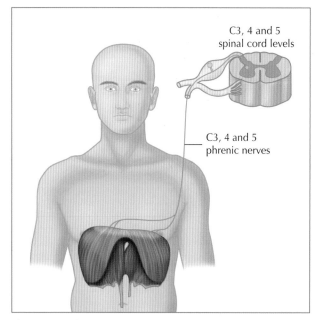

C3, 4 and 5
spinal cord levels

C3, 4 and 5
phrenic nerves

Figure 3.2: *Phrenic nerve innervation of the diaphragm.*

Furthermore, C1–2 supply the rectus capitis lateralis and anterior, C1–3 the longus capitis, C2–3 the sternocleidomastoid, and C3–4 the trapezius. The levator scapulae and medial fibers of the scalenes are also supplied via the cervical plexus.

Sensory Branches

The sensory (cutaneous) supply of the cervical plexus serves the skin of the neck, scalp, ear, and upper thorax, and comprises the following nerves (C1 has no skin sensory distribution):

- Great auricular nerve
- Lesser occipital nerve
- Transverse cervical nerve
- Supraclavicular nerve

All the above nerves penetrate a small area on the neck known as *Erb's point*, named after the German neurologist Wilhelm Heinrich Erb. This point is located posteriorly to the middle aspect of the sternocleidomastoid muscle, and this specific location on the neck is commonly used for cervical plexus nerve blocks in preparation for head or neck surgery (Figure 3.3).

Great Auricular Nerve
The great auricular nerve is the largest ascending branch of the plexus and originates from C2 and C3. It provides sensory supply to the outer ear and also to the skin overlying the angle of the jaw.

Lesser Occipital Nerve
The lesser occipital nerve originates mainly from C2 and supplies the sensation to the superior posterior aspect of the scalp.

Transverse Cervical Nerve
The transverse cervical nerve originates from C2 and C3, and, as its name suggests, it traverses the sternocleidomastoid. The nerve supplies the sensation for the anterior aspect of the neck and sternum.

Supraclavicular Nerve
The supraclavicular nerve originates from C3 and C4 and supplies sensation to the skin overlying the supraclavicular fossa (above the clavicle) and also to the sternoclavicular joint.

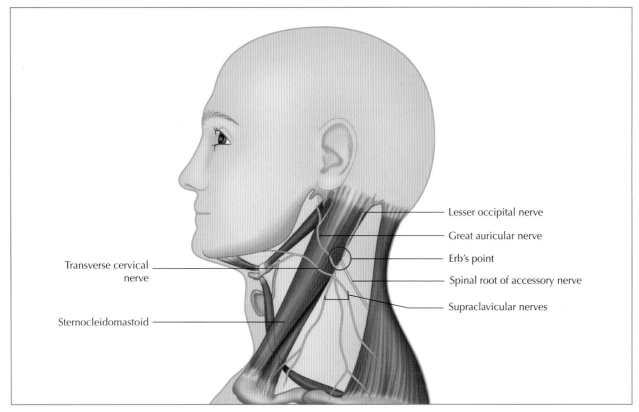

Figure 3.3: *Erb's point location for cervical plexus nerve block.*

■ Brachial Plexus

The brachial plexus (Figure 3.4) is composed of nerves emanating from the spinal cord at a vertebral level (C1–C4, C5–T1). The brachial plexus passes through the space formed between the scalenus anterior and scalenus medius muscles, and is known as the *interscalene triangle*.

The nerve roots of C5 and C6 join to form the *upper trunk*, while the nerve roots of C8 and T1 join to form the *lower trunk*. C7 does not join with any other nerve root; it alone makes up the *middle trunk*. As the trunks pass beneath the clavicle, they then divide again into six sections: three anterior divisions and three posterior divisions. From here, they continue to form three cords: medial, lateral, and posterior, around the axillary artery. The upper and lower trunks contribute to the middle trunk and all three trunks contribute to the formation of the *posterior cord*. The middle trunk, in turn, sends a contribution with C5 and C6 to form the *lateral cord*. The two remaining nerves, C8 and T1, form the *medial cord*.

The branches now continue and emerge from the cords. The lateral cord sends one branch to become the *musculocutaneous nerve*. The other branch of the lateral

cord joins with a branch from the medial cord to form the *median nerve*. The second branch of the medial cord becomes the *ulnar nerve*, and the posterior cord becomes the *axillary nerve* and the *radial nerve*.

It makes perfect sense in this chapter to cover the peripheral nerves that exit from the brachial plexus (Figure 3.5), and to focus a little bit more on their anatomy, sensory, and motor function. Subsequently, the discussion will move on to how to assess these nerves, hopefully without making it too complex to understand—neurological testing can be a difficult subject to get your head around. However, I do not think it has to be that difficult if it is taught in a straightforward way. I will try my best to explain this fascinating subject simply.

In this section, I would like to discuss the five terminal branches (peripheral nerves) of the brachial plexus, namely:

1. Radial nerve
2. Median nerve
3. Ulnar nerve
4. Musculocutaneous nerve
5. Axillary nerve

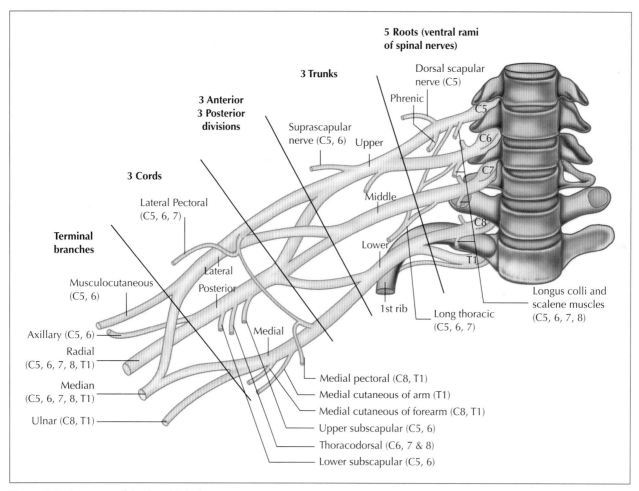

Figure 3.4: *Anatomy of the brachial plexus.*

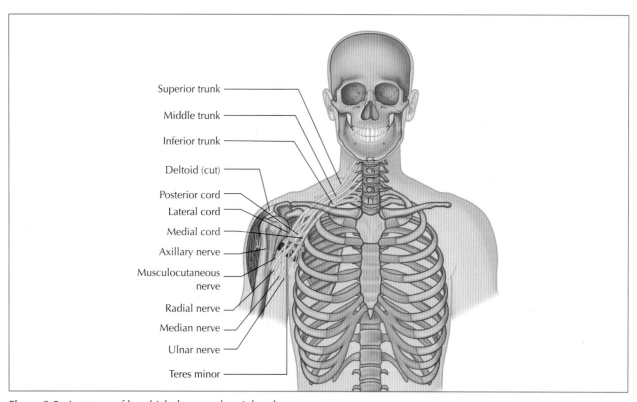

Figure 3.5: *Anatomy of brachial plexus and peripheral nerves.*

Brachial plexus explained on whiteboard

Brachial plexus—PowerPoint

Brachial plexus branches explained on whiteboard

Brachial plexus branches— PowerPoint

Radial Nerve

The posterior cord of the brachial plexus from the specific root levels of C5–8 and T1 forms the *radial nerve*, as shown in Figure 3.6, passes through the posterior axillary wall to reach deltoid and teres minor, follows the brachial artery in the arm, and innervates the triceps muscle. The radial nerve continues and passes over the lateral epicondyle and through the cubital fossa, and then divides into the deep (posterior interosseous nerve) and superficial branches.

In terms of motor function, the radial nerve initially supplies all three heads of the triceps muscles, before continuing its journey into the forearm and hand. However, Rezzouk et al. (2004) found, through 20 cadaver dissections, that the long head of the triceps muscle was innervated by the axillary nerve, and none of the heads were supplied by the radial nerve.

Motor Supply

The radial nerve provides motor innervation to the following muscles, as shown in Figure 3.7:

- Triceps
- Anconeus
- Brachioradialis
- Extensor carpi radialis longus

The deep branch of the radial nerve supplies:

- Extensor carpi radialis brevis
- Supinator

The posterior interosseous nerve (deep branch continued) innervates:

- Extensor digitorum
- Extensor digiti minimi
- Extensor carpi ulnaris
- Extensor pollicis longus
- Extensor pollicis brevis
- Extensor indicis
- Abductor pollicis longus

Sensory Supply

The *sensory* component is provided mainly by the posterior cutaneous nerve, which supplies a strip of skin down the center of the back of the forearm and also the

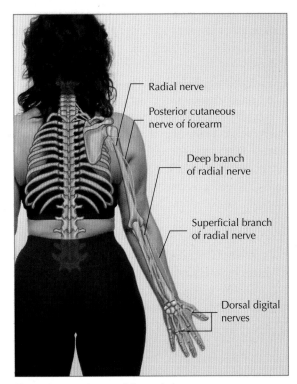

Radial nerve

Posterior cutaneous nerve of forearm

Deep branch of radial nerve

Superficial branch of radial nerve

Dorsal digital nerves

Figure 3.6: *Pathway of the radial nerve.*

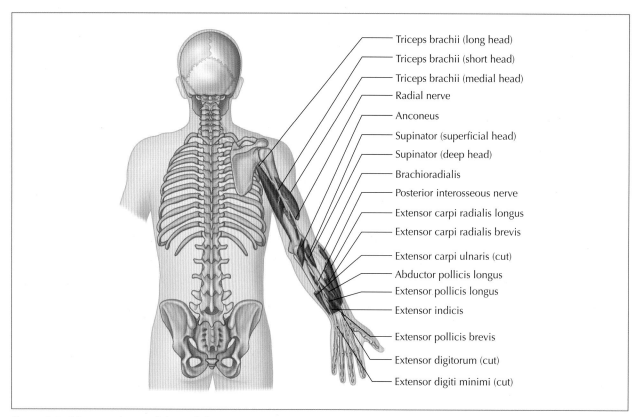

Triceps brachii (long head)
Triceps brachii (short head)
Triceps brachii (medial head)
Radial nerve
Anconeus
Supinator (superficial head)
Supinator (deep head)
Brachioradialis
Posterior interosseous nerve
Extensor carpi radialis longus
Extensor carpi radialis brevis
Extensor carpi ulnaris (cut)
Abductor pollicis longus
Extensor pollicis longus
Extensor indicis
Extensor pollicis brevis
Extensor digitorum (cut)
Extensor digiti minimi (cut)

Figure 3.7: *Motor pathway of the radial nerve.*

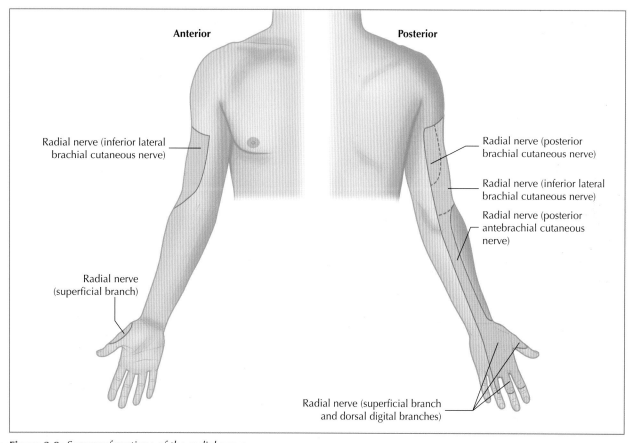

Anterior   Posterior

Radial nerve (inferior lateral
brachial cutaneous nerve)

Radial nerve (posterior
brachial cutaneous nerve)

Radial nerve (inferior lateral
brachial cutaneous nerve)

Radial nerve (posterior
antebrachial cutaneous
nerve)

Radial nerve
(superficial branch)

Radial nerve (superficial branch
and dorsal digital branches)

Figure 3.8: *Sensory functions of the radial nerve.*

elbow joint. The superficial branch provides sensory innervation to the dorsal surface of the hand and the lateral three and a half fingers, short of the nail beds, as well as to the web space between the thumb and the index finger (Figure 3.8).

Any form of trauma to the radial nerve may result in motor weakness in supination and/or extension of the wrist (wrist drop) and in extension of the fingers. There may be sensory loss to the posterior forearm, radial side of the forearm, and the dorsal aspect of the three and a half digits (excluding the nail beds), and also to the web space between the thumb and the index finger.

Radial Nerve Strength Test

To ascertain the motor contractibility of the radial nerve, the patient resists against an applied force using the muscle of their thumb (extensor pollicis longus), as shown in Figure 3.9.

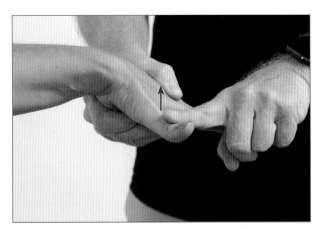

Figure 3.9: *Radial nerve strength assessment through contraction of the extensor pollicis longus.*

Radial nerve testing

Median Nerve

The *median nerve* originates from the lateral (C5, C6) and medial (C8, T1) cords of the brachial plexus, as well as having a branch from the middle trunk (C7) (which continues to the lateral cord). The nerve proceeds through the axilla and lateral to the brachial artery, and lies between the brachialis and biceps brachii muscles. It then passes over the brachial artery, and so is situated medially as it

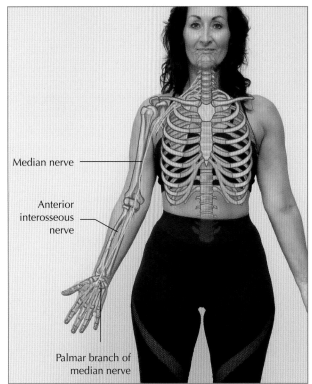

Median nerve

Anterior interosseous nerve

Palmar branch of median nerve

Figure 3.10: *Pathway of the median nerve.*

continues its journey toward the cubital fossa; here it gives off an articular branch to the elbow joint (Figure 3.10).

The median nerve continues through the two heads of the pronator teres muscle and lies between the two muscles of the flexor superficialis profundus (FDP) and flexor digitorum superficialis (FDS), and now gives rise to two main branches in the forearm called the *anterior interosseous nerve*, which supplies the deep muscles in the forearm, and the *palmar cutaneous nerve*, which innervates the skin of the lateral palm. The median nerve then enters the hand through the carpal tunnel, where it terminates by dividing into two branches called the *recurrent branch*, which supplies the thenar muscles, and the *palmar digital branch*, which innervates the sensory supply to the palmar surface, the thumb, index finger, and half the ring finger.

Motor Supply

The median nerve innervates the following muscles (Figure 3.11) in different layers:

Superficial layer:

- Pronator teres
- Flexor carpi radialis
- Palmaris longus

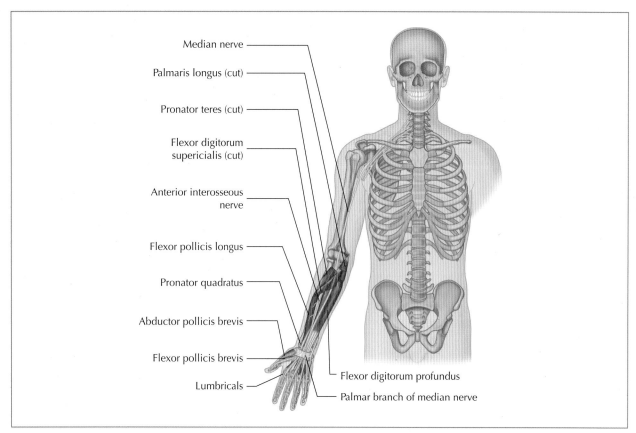

Median nerve

Palmaris longus (cut)

Pronator teres (cut)

Flexor digitorum supericialis (cut)

Anterior interosseous nerve

Flexor pollicis longus

Pronator quadratus

Abductor pollicis brevis

Flexor pollicis brevis

Lumbricals

Flexor digitorum profundus

Palmar branch of median nerve

Figure 3.11: *Motor pathway of the median nerve.*

Intermediate layer:

- Flexor digitorum superficialis

Deep layer:

- Flexor digitorum profundus (lateral half)
- Flexor pollicis longus
- Pronator quadratus

Hand Muscles

The muscles listed below make up part of the thenar eminence and control movements of the thumb (pollex). They are called the *LOAF muscles* (Figure 3.12), while the last three are known as the *OAF muscles*.

- **L**ateral lumbricals (first and second)
- **O**pponens pollicis
- **A**bductor pollicis brevis
- **F**lexor pollicis brevis

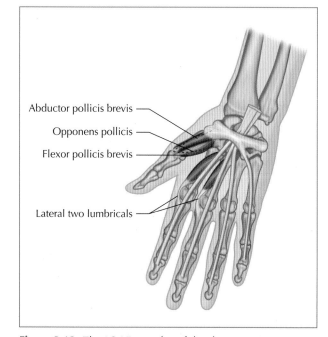

Abductor pollicis brevis

Opponens pollicis

Flexor pollicis brevis

Lateral two lumbricals

Figure 3.12: *The LOAF muscles of the thenar eminence.*

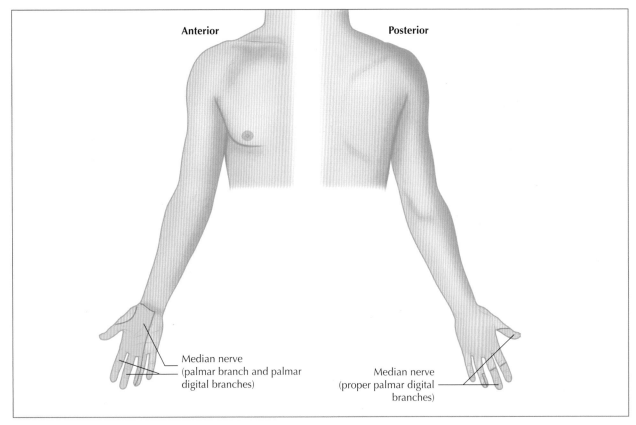

Figure 3.13: *Sensory functions of the median nerve.*

Sensory Supply

The median nerve provides the sensory supply for the palmar surface of the thenar eminence, the thumb, and the index, middle, and half the ring fingers, as well as the associated nail beds (Figure 3.13).

Median Nerve Strength Test—Pinch Grip

The patient pinches their thumb and index finger, as shown in Figure 3.14. The patient is then asked to resist the motion of the therapist trying to separate the patient's thumb and finger.

Trauma to the median nerve normally occurs within the carpal tunnel, producing the well-known affliction *carpal tunnel syndrome* (CTS). CTS is commonly caused by swelling of the tendon sheath (tenosynovitis) as a result of repetitive motion of the fingers (e.g., typing) and also thickened ligaments. In extreme cases, the thenar eminence muscles (LOAF) will atrophy (waste away) because of the compression of the nerve. The median nerve can also be damaged at the elbow through a supracondylar fracture, which will lead to paralysis of the flexors and pronators in the forearm, with an appearance of permanent supination. Carpal tunnel syndrome can be distinguished from other median nerve lesions by the

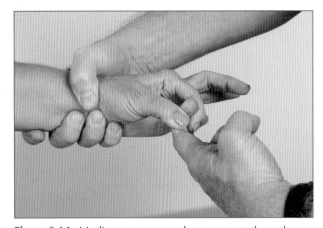

Figure 3.14: *Median nerve strength assessment through a pinch grip test.*

lack of loss of sensation over the thenar eminence as the palmar cutaneous branch is not lost.

Median nerve testing & carpal tunnel syndrome

Ulnar Nerve

The *ulnar nerve* (C8, T1) initially originates from the spinal roots of C8 and T1 and forms the medial cords. The nerve continues its journey medially down the arm toward the elbow, and passes posterior to the medial epicondyle of the humerus (the nerve is palpable in this area and is a common site for injury). It continues in the forearm and penetrates the two heads of the flexor carpi ulnaris muscle, before traveling along the ulna bone. Upon reaching the wrist, the nerve continues through the tunnel of Guyon, or Guyon's canal (located between the pisiform and hamate bones of the wrist and superficial to the carpal tunnel), and terminates in the superficial and deep branches (Figure 3.15).

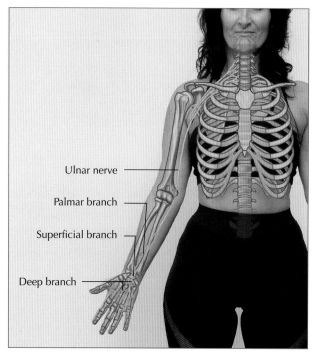

Figure 3.15: *Pathway of the ulnar nerve.*

Motor Supply

The ulnar nerve innervates the following muscles, as shown in Figure 3.16:

Forearm:

- Flexor carpi ulnaris
- Flexor superficialis profundus (medial half)

Hand Muscles

The muscles below make up the hypothenar eminence (OAF) and control the movements of the little finger (digiti minimi), as shown in Figure 3.17:

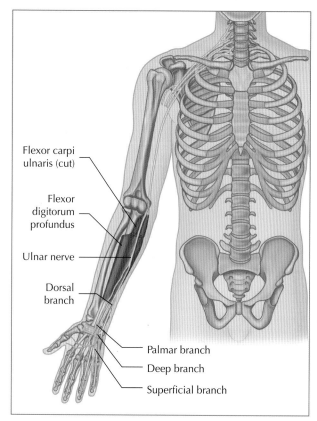

Figure 3.16: *Motor pathway of the ulnar nerve.*

- Opponens digiti minimi
- Abductor digiti minimi
- Flexor digiti minimi brevis

The ulnar nerve also supplies the following muscles of the hand:

- Medial two lumbricals
- Adductor pollicis
- Palmaris brevis
- Interossei

Sensory Supply

The ulnar nerve innervates the medial side of the palm and the corresponding medial dorsal surface, as well as the little finger and half the ring finger (Figure 3.18).

Ulnar Nerve Strength Test

To ascertain the motor contractibility of the ulnar nerve, the patient resists abduction of the little finger (abductor digiti minimi), as shown in Figure 3.19.

Damage to the ulnar nerve is common at the medial epicondyle of the elbow because of its susceptibility. The nerve can be compressed within the cubital tunnel,

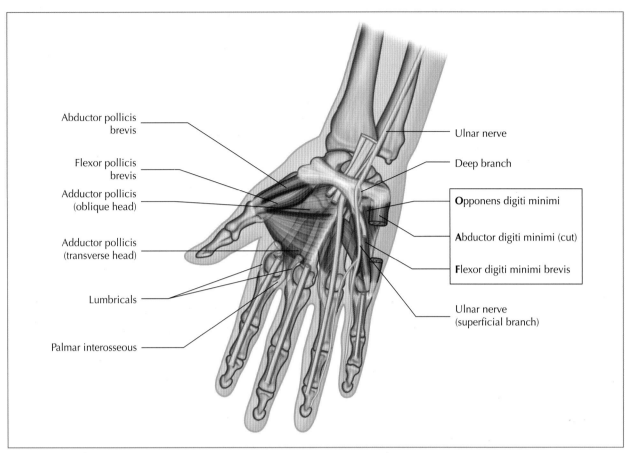

Abductor pollicis brevis

Flexor pollicis brevis

Adductor pollicis (oblique head)

Adductor pollicis (transverse head)

Lumbricals

Palmar interosseous

Ulnar nerve

Deep branch

Opponens digiti minimi

Abductor digiti minimi (cut)

Flexor digiti minimi brevis

Ulnar nerve (superficial branch)

Figure 3.17: *The OAF muscles of the hypothenar eminence (boxed).*

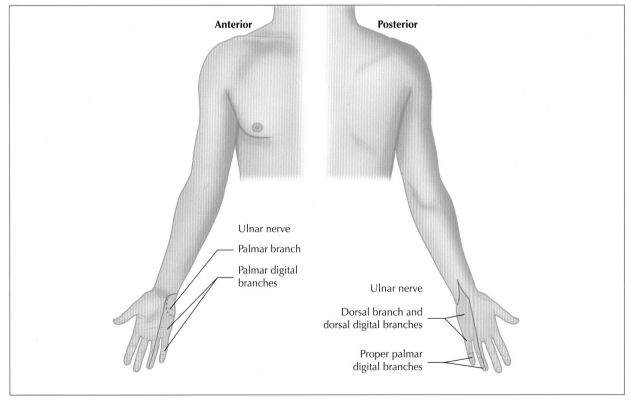

Anterior

Posterior

Ulnar nerve

Palmar branch

Palmar digital branches

Ulnar nerve

Dorsal branch and dorsal digital branches

Proper palmar digital branches

Figure 3.18: *Sensory functions of the ulnar nerve.*

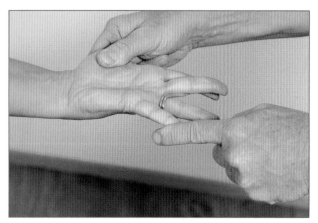

Figure 3.19: *Ulnar nerve strength assessment through abduction of the little finger.*

leading to an affliction known as *cubital tunnel syndrome.* It can also be stretched or even compressed within the hand, which commonly occurs in or near to the tunnel of Guyon; this is especially the case in cyclists, because the hand is in an extended and ulnar-deviated position, causing stretching of the nerve through the tunnel. In extreme cases, the fingers are unable to abduct and adduct, and movement of the little finger and ring finger will be reduced; a loss of sensation will be experienced in the area of the ulnar nerve innervation.

 **Ulnar nerve testing**

Musculocutaneous Nerve

The *musculocutaneous nerve* is formed from the terminal branch of the lateral cord of the brachial plexus (C5, C6, and C7). The nerve continues its journey down the arm and innervates the coracobrachialis and then the brachialis and biceps brachii (Figure 3.20). It then passes lateral to the tendon of the biceps, before entering the forearm to supply the necessary sensory innervation to the lateral forearm as the lateral cutaneous nerve.

Motor Supply
The musculocutaneous nerve innervates:

- Coracobrachialis
- Brachialis
- Biceps brachii

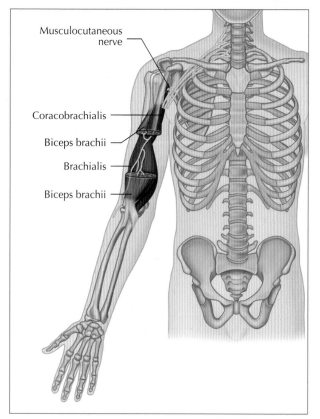

Figure 3.20: *Motor pathway of the musculocutaneous nerve.*

Sensory Supply
Sensory supply is through the lateral cutaneous nerve, which innervates the area of the skin on the lateral part of the forearm (Figure 3.21).

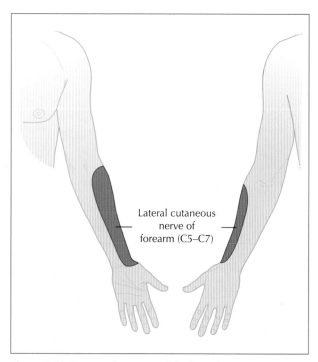

Figure 3.21: *Sensory functions of the lateral cutaneous nerve.*

Damage to the musculocutaneous nerve is very rare because it is fairly well protected, and so there is no need to discuss any injuries to this nerve.

Axillary Nerve

The C5–6 spinal nerve root travels along the upper trunk and connects to the posterior cord. The *axillary nerve* is a branch of the posterior cord and located within the region of the axilla, posterior to the axillary artery and anterior to the subscapularis. The nerve then divides into two branches called the *posterior terminal branch*, which supplies the teres minor muscle, and the *anterior terminal branch*, which supplies the deltoid muscle (Figure 3.22).

Motor Supply

The axillary nerve innervates:

- Deltoid
- Teres minor

Sensory Supply

Sensory supply is through the posterior terminal branch, which innervates the skin region inferior to the deltoid muscle (Figure 3.23), a small autonomous area known as the *regimental badge* because of the usual location of

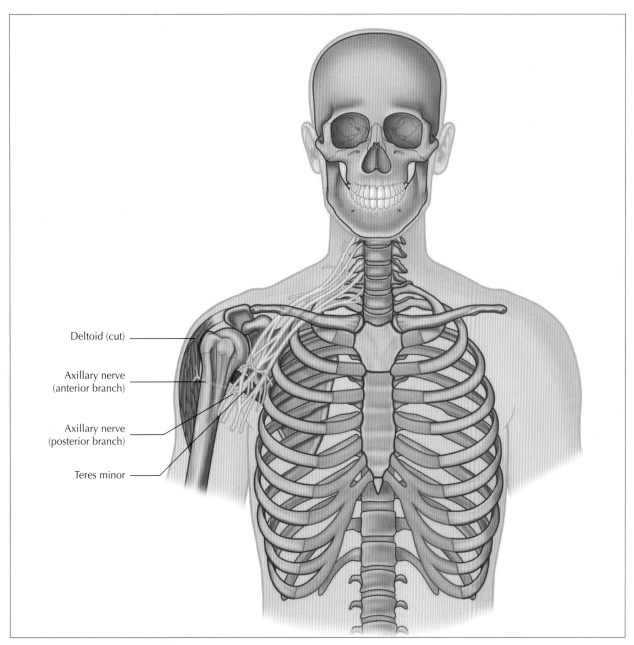

Deltoid (cut)

Axillary nerve (anterior branch)

Axillary nerve (posterior branch)

Teres minor

Figure 3.22: *Motor pathway of the axillary nerve.*

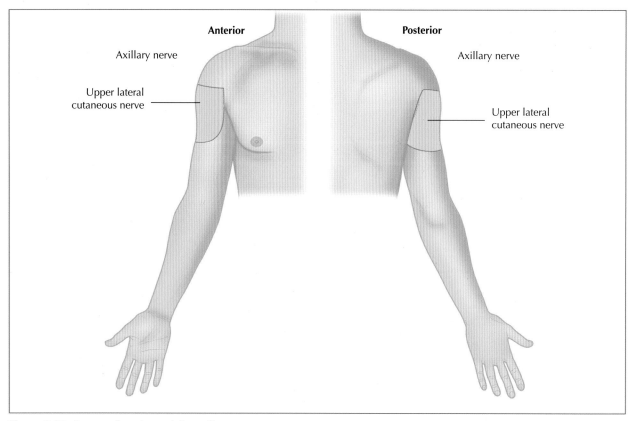

Figure 3.23: *Sensory functions of the axillary nerve.*

sergeant stripes or badge on the upper arm of a military uniform (Figure 3.24).

Damage to the axillary nerve is normally through dislocation of the glenohumeral joint or a fracture to the surgical neck of the humerus, with subsequent atrophy of the deltoid and teres minor muscles to the extent that the acromion process and the greater tubercle of the humerus can be seen and easily palpated. Shoulder abduction will be weak and difficult, and sensory loss will be to the "regimental badge" area.

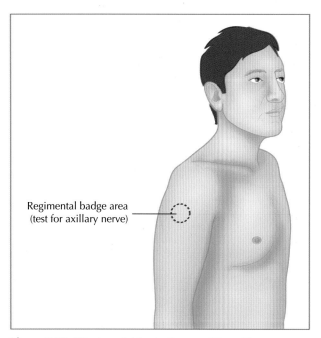

Figure 3.24: *"Regimental badge" area of the axillary nerve.*

Axillary nerve testing

Brachial plexus branches explained on whiteboard

Brachial plexus branches— PowerPoint

4

Anatomy and Function of the Lumbosacral Plexus

Even though I will mention the lumbosacral plexus, I feel it makes perfect sense to individualize each of the plexuses, namely the *lumbar plexus* and the *sacral plexus*, and to discuss them separately. I personally believe that this is a better way of learning the nerves associated with the areas of the lumbar and sacral spines.

■ Lumbar Plexus

The *lumbar plexus* (Figure 4.1) forms the upper part of the lumbosacral plexus, and is formed by the divisions of the first four lumbar nerves (L1–4) and the subcostal nerve (T12).

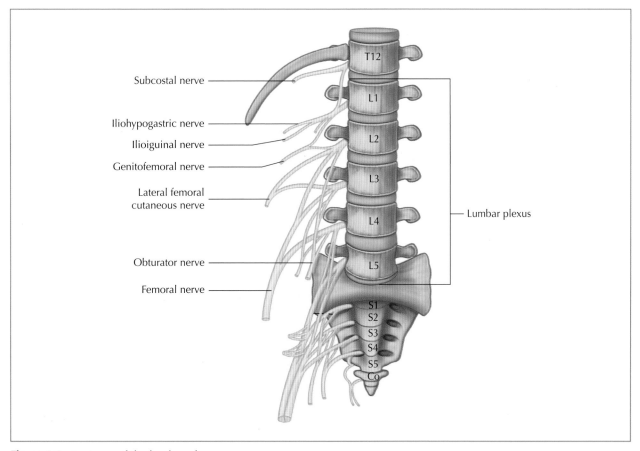

Figure 4.1: *Anatomy of the lumbar plexus.*

Branches of nerves of the lumber plexus include:

- Ilioinguinal and iliohypogastric nerves
- Genitofemoral nerve
- Lateral femoral cutaneous nerve
- Femoral nerve
- Obturator nerve

Ilioinguinal and Iliohypogastric Nerves

The first lumbar segment, L1, forms the *ilioinguinal* and *iliohypogastric* nerves (Figure 4.2), which innervate the conjoint tendon only of the internal oblique and transversus abdominis muscles.

The *ilioinguinal nerve*, from a sensory perspective, supplies the skin over the root of the penis and the upper part of the scrotum (in males), and the skin over the labia majora and mons pubis (in females).

The *iliohypogastric nerve* basically supplies the skin over the pubis region and innervates the lateral gluteal area; it then subdivides into the lateral and anterior cutaneous branches. The *lateral cutaneous branch* supplies the skin over the gluteal area, while the *anterior cutaneous branch* supplies an area over the pubis called the *hypogastric region*.

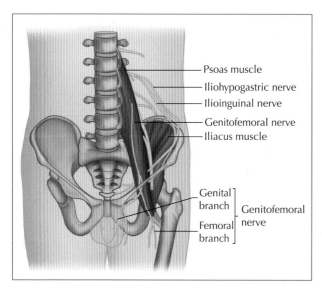

Figure 4.2: *Ilioinguinal and Iliohypogastric nerve anatomy.*

Genitofemoral Nerve

The *genitofemoral nerve*, which is formed from L1 and L2, pierces the psoas major muscle, and subdivides into the genital and femoral branches (Figure 4.3). The *genital*

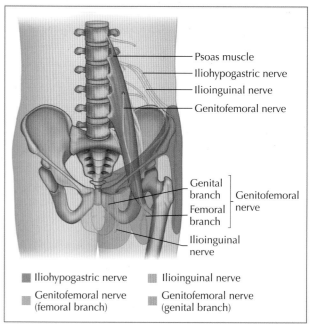

Figure 4.3: *Ilioinguinal, iliohypogastric, and genitofemoral nerve innervation.*

branch enters the deep inguinal ring and supplies the skin of the scrotal region and the cremaster muscle (elevates the testes in males); in women, this branch supplies the area over the pubis and labia majora. The *femoral branch* supplies the area of the skin on the upper, anterior, and medial aspects of the thigh.

It would make sense to briefly discuss the *cremasteric reflex* (Figure 4.4)—a reflex found only in males.

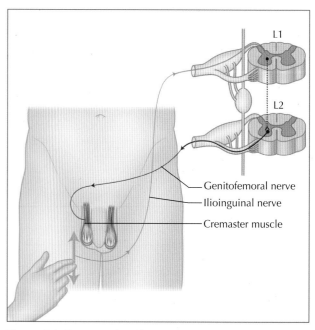

Figure 4.4: *Cremasteric reflex.*

It occurs by lightly touching the inner thigh, to which the normal response is an immediate contraction of the cremaster muscle, causing an elevation of the testis on the corresponding side. This happens because the sensory component of the ilioinguinal nerve is activated, leading to the contraction of the cremaster muscle through the motor supply of the genitofemoral nerve.

Lateral Femoral Cutaneous Nerve

The *lateral femoral cutaneous nerve* (Figure 4.5) originates from levels L2–3 and passes directly over the iliacus muscle and under the inguinal ligament. It then continues over the sartorius muscle and supplies the skin on the anterior and lateral aspects of the thigh.

There is a medical condition, called *meralgia paresthetica*, that relates to a compression of the lateral femoral cutaneous nerve. (The lateral femoral cutaneous nerve often passes through the inguinal ligament and it is suggested that because of this it can become damaged and lead to meralgia paraesthetica.) This typically affects people who put on weight over time and their underwear garments become increasingly tighter; it is also seen in pregnant women because, as the fetus grows, the increased

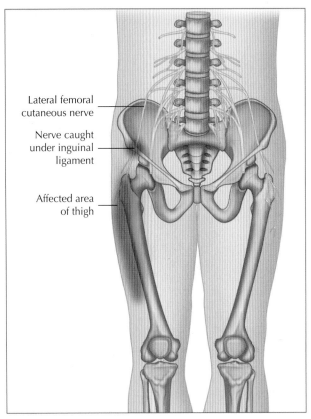

Figure 4.6: *Meralgia paresthetica and the inguinal ligament area where the nerve gets compressed.*

size of the abdomen can cause pressure to the nerve as it passes under the lateral side of the inguinal ligament, adjacent to the ASIS (see Figure 4.6). The condition is also nicknamed *skinny pants syndrome*, which relates to teenagers wearing skin-tight jeans.

Femoral Nerve

The *femoral nerve* (Figure 4.7), the largest branch of the lumbar plexus, is located in the thigh and not in the leg as some texts claim. It originates from the dorsal divisions of the ventral rami of the second, third, and fourth lumbar nerves (L2–4).

In the femoral region, the nerve subdivides into the anterior and posterior divisions, and supplies the following muscles, as shown in Figure 4.8, before subdividing further into many smaller branches throughout the anterior and medial thigh:

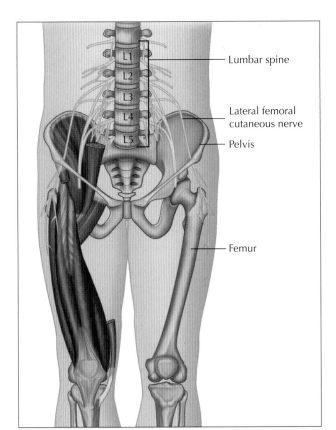

Figure 4.5: *Lateral femoral cutaneous nerve anatomy.*

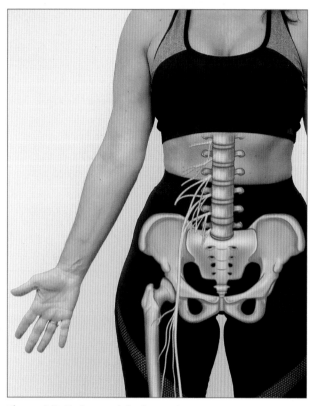

Figure 4.7: *Pathway of the femoral nerve.*

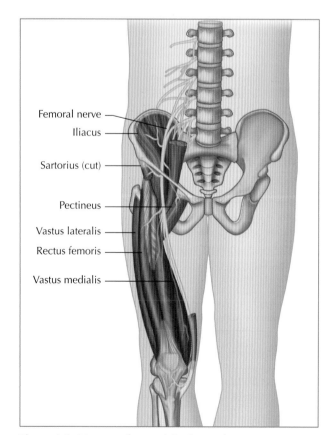

Femoral nerve
Iliacus
Sartorius (cut)
Pectineus
Vastus lateralis
Rectus femoris
Vastus medialis

Figure 4.8: *Motor pathway of the femoral nerve.*

The *anterior division* innervates:

- Iliacus
- Sartorius
- Pectineus

The *posterior division* innervates:

- Rectus femoris
- Vastus lateralis
- Vastus medialis
- Vastus intermedius

The cutaneous branch of the femoral nerve has two branches: one called the *anterior femoral cutaneous branch*, which innervates the anterior thigh, and the other called the *saphenous nerve*. The saphenous nerve is the longest sensory (cutaneous) component of the femoral nerve and supplies sensation to the medial side of the lower leg and foot (Figure 4.9). Because of its significance

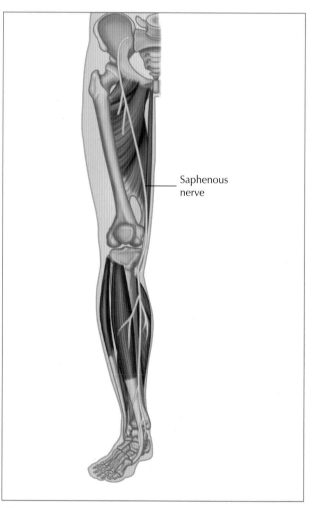

Saphenous nerve

Figure 4.9: *Saphenous nerve and its innervation of the lower leg.*

and its common pathway with the returning saphenous vein, the saphenous nerve is commonly damaged during the procedure in which the vein is removed for use in bypass surgery; the nerve can also be damaged during knee surgery.

Obturator Nerve

The *obturator nerve* (Figure 4.10) originates from the ventral divisions of the second, third, and fourth lumbar nerves (L2, L3, L4) in the lumbar plexus, and passes through the obturator foramen. The nerve innervates:

- Obturator externus
- Pectineus (occasionally)
- Adductor brevis
- Half of adductor magnus
- Adductor longus
- Gracilis

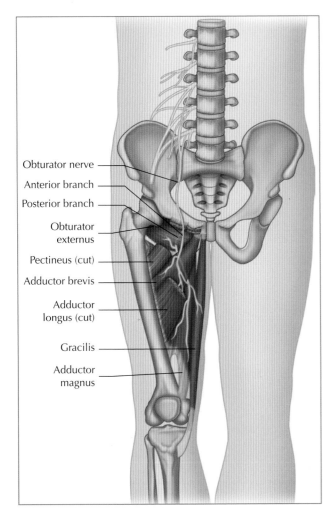

Figure 4.10: *Motor pathway of the obturator nerve.*

Despite its name, the obturator nerve is not responsible for the innervation of the obturator internus muscle; this muscle is supplied by the obturator internus nerve (L5–S2) from the sciatic nerve roots.

The cutaneous supply of the obturator nerve is to the area of the medial thigh.

CASE STUDY 4.1

I find it particularly interesting when someone comes into the clinic with knee pain, especially when they can do most of their exercises without exacerbating the symptoms. In general, I am of the belief that if you have knee pain, then most movements involving bending and extending (such as squatting, lunging, and walking up and down stairs) should cause irritation. If these particular movements do not irritate, then maybe the knee pain is a symptom and not the actual causative factor. This is very true in the case of the following patient. Over many weeks, a friend of mine would always mention that his right knee was hurting, but he could not say which particular movements caused the pain to increase. He simply said, "It just hurts most of the time without actually doing anything."

In terms of the assessment, I went through all my typical knee-testing procedures, and none of the movements seemed to cause any increase in his symptoms. Next, I decided to assess his hip joint; again, I did not find anything of particular concern, although his right hip was a little stiffer than his left. I then proceeded to assess his lumbar spine and I found the vertebral motion between L3–4 to be restricted compared with the levels above and below. I decided to mobilize this area and also included some soft-tissue techniques for his paravertebral muscles, finishing with a manipulation at the L3–4 level. To be honest, the symptoms did not change very much initially, because he still spoke about his knee pain. With a combination of soft-tissue, hip-mobility, and spinal-manipulation techniques, however, the patient started to respond, and after approximately four to six treatments, the knee pain finally subsided.

Sacral Plexus

The *sacral plexus* (Figure 4.11) is basically the lower part of the lumbosacral plexus and is a branching network of

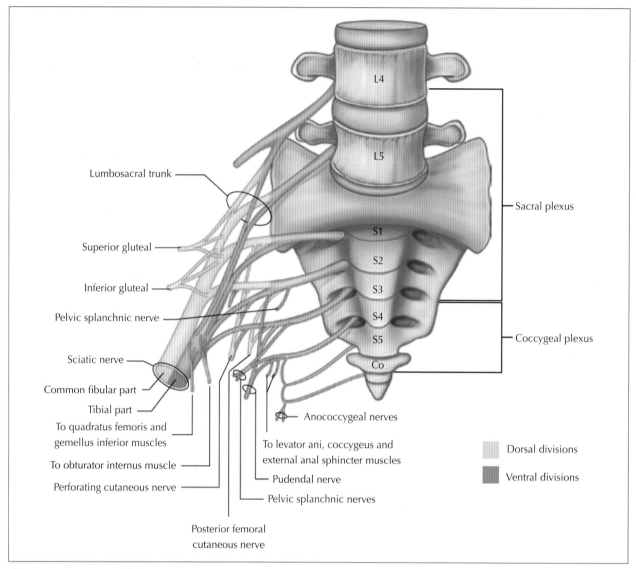

Figure 4.11: *Anatomy of the sacral plexus.*

nerves that provides motor and sensory supply to part of the pelvis, the posterior thigh, most of the lower leg, and the entire foot. It makes up part of the larger lumbosacral plexus. The sacral plexus is formed from the anterior rami of the spinal nerves L4, L5, S1, S2, S3, and S4, and each of these anterior rami gives rise to anterior and posterior branches. The *anterior branches* supply the flexor muscles of the lower limb, and the *posterior branches* supply the extensor and abductor muscles.

All the nerve roots entering the sacral plexus split into anterior and posterior divisions. The nerves arising from these divisions are:

- Sciatic nerve:
  - tibial nerve: L4–S3
  - common fibular nerve: L4–S2
- Superior gluteal nerve: L4–S1

- Inferior gluteal nerve: L5–S2
- Posterior femoral cutaneous nerve: S1–S3
- Pudendal nerve: S2–S4
- Nerve to quadratus femoris and gemellus inferior: L4–S1
- Nerve to obturator internus and gemellus superior: L5–S2
- Nerve to piriformis: S1–2

Sciatic Nerve

The *sciatic nerve* (Figure 4.12) is by far the longest and widest nerve in the human body. It is formed from the upper sacral plexus of the anterior primary rami of L4, L5, S1, S2, and S3. It travels out of the greater sciatic foramen, normally passing inferior to the piriformis muscle (Figure 4.13).

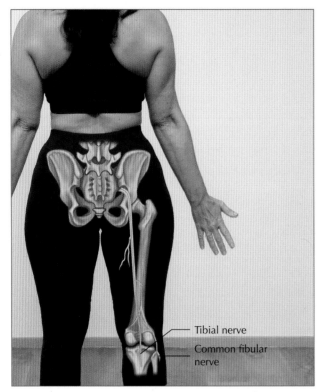

Figure 4.12: *Pathway of the sciatic nerve.*

The sciatic nerve innervates the following muscles, as shown by Figure 4.14:

- Biceps femoris
- Semimembranosus
- Semitendinosus
- Half of adductor magnus

True sciatic nerve damage can result in altered sensation, numbness, weakness, and pain. Depending on the source and level of irritation, the pain can be mild to severe. Sciatic nerve irritation usually occurs at the L5 or S1 level of the spine, and only on one side. Pain can travel all the way to the foot and affect normal motion, but with normal healing, the referred pain should dissipate and become more centralized. Unresolved chronic pain, especially of unknown origin, should be brought to the attention of the medical doctor or primary healthcare team.

At approximately mid-thigh, the sciatic nerve subdivides into the *tibial nerve* and the *common fibular nerve* (also known as the *common peroneal nerve*).

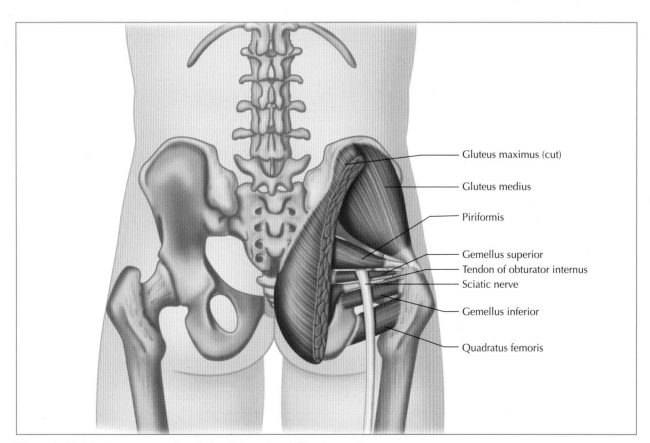

Figure 4.13: *Sciatic nerve and the relationship to the piriformis muscle.*

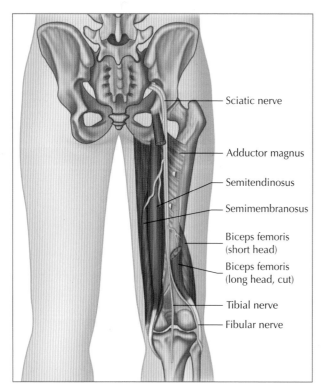

Figure 4.14: *Motor pathway of the sciatic nerve.*

Tibial Nerve

Along with the common fibular nerve, the tibial nerve (Figure 4.15) originates proximal to the popliteal fossa as a major branch of the sciatic nerve, and innervates the muscles of the posterior compartment of the leg:

- Gastrocnemius
- Soleus
- Plantaris
- Popliteus
- Tibialis posterior
- Flexor digitorum longus
- Flexor hallucis longus

One of the lower branches of the tibial nerve becomes the *medial plantar nerve* of the foot (Figure 4.16) and innervates:

- Abductor hallucis
- Flexor digitorum brevis
- Flexor hallucis brevis
- First lumbrical

The other lower branch becomes the *lateral plantar nerve* and innervates:

- Abductor digiti minimi
- Quadratus plantae

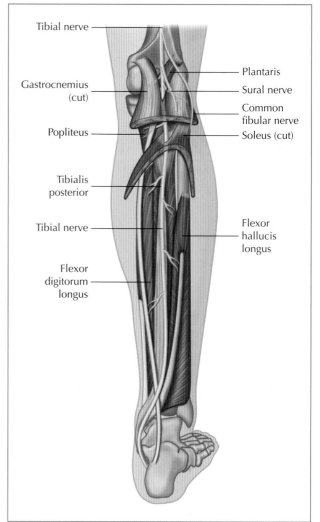

Figure 4.15: *Motor pathway of the tibial nerve.*

- Adductor hallucis
- Flexor digiti minimi brevis
- Plantar interossei
- Dorsal interossei
- Three lateral lumbricals

Common Fibular Nerve

The *common fibular nerve*, shown in Figure 4.17, originates, via the sciatic nerve, from the dorsal branches of the fourth and fifth lumbar nerves (L4–5) and the first and second sacral nerves (S1–2). It divides into the *superficial fibular nerve* and the *deep fibular nerve*.

The *superficial fibular nerve* innervates:

- Fibularis longus
- Fibularis brevis

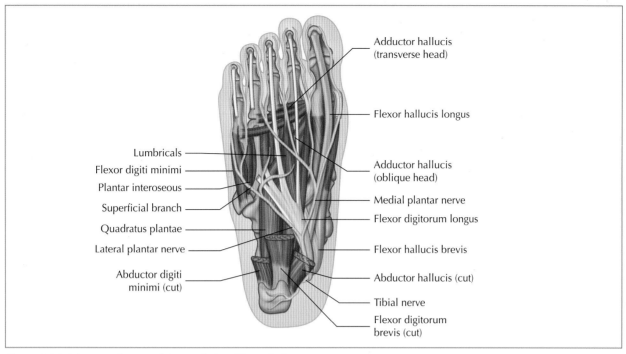

Labels:
- Adductor hallucis (transverse head)
- Flexor hallucis longus
- Lumbricals
- Flexor digiti minimi
- Plantar interoseous
- Superficial branch
- Quadratus plantae
- Lateral plantar nerve
- Abductor digiti minimi (cut)
- Adductor hallucis (oblique head)
- Medial plantar nerve
- Flexor digitorum longus
- Flexor hallucis brevis
- Abductor hallucis (cut)
- Tibial nerve
- Flexor digitorum brevis (cut)

Figure 4.16: *Motor pathways of the medial and lateral plantar nerves.*

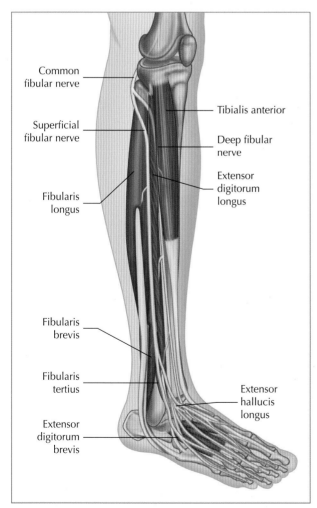

Labels:
- Common fibular nerve
- Superficial fibular nerve
- Fibularis longus
- Fibularis brevis
- Fibularis tertius
- Extensor digitorum brevis
- Tibialis anterior
- Deep fibular nerve
- Extensor digitorum longus
- Extensor hallucis longus

Figure 4.17: *Motor pathway of the common fibular nerve.*

The *deep fibular nerve* innervates:

- Tibialis anterior
- Extensor digitorum longus (EDL)
- Fibularis tertius
- Extensor hallucis longus (EHL)
- Extensor hallucis brevis
- Extensor digitorum brevis

Sural Nerve

There is also a sensory branch of the tibial nerve called the *medial cutaneous nerve* and a branch of the common fibular nerve called the *lateral sural cutaneous nerve.* Together, these make up the *sural nerve* (Latin *sura* = "calf of the leg"), which is located in the calf region and supplies the sensation to the skin of the lateral foot and lateral lower ankle, as shown in Figure 4.18.

CASE STUDY 4.2

This is an interesting case of a 50-year-old male who telephoned me one day and said that he could not extend his left great toe, and also that he was unable to lift (dorsiflex) his ankle fully, as it felt very weak. He said he had been told he has a condition called *drop foot* (see "Drop Foot" section in Chapter 10), and the doctors diagnosed the problem to be coming from a disc in his lower spine affecting the L5 nerve root. The patient

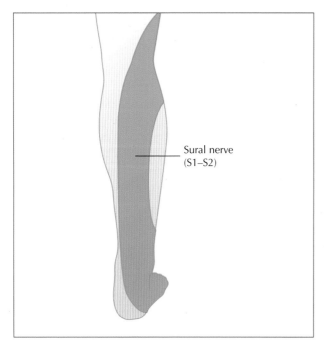

Figure 4.18: *Sural nerve innervation.*

Sural nerve (S1–S2)

categorically stated that he did not think his back was the problem, because he had never suffered from any type of back pain.

On the phone, he mentioned something about his left leg and an issue below his knee, but was a little vague, so I decided to investigate this a little further during the initial consultation. The patient was booked in for an MRI of his lumbar spine, so I decided to wait for the results before I saw him. The findings were all negative with regard to anything spinal related that could be responsible for his symptoms; the doctors were now confused and unable to suggest anything as the underlying cause of his drop foot.

When I assessed him, I did not find anything wrong with his lumbar spine; furthermore, the L4, L5, and S1 reflexes were normal, at 2++ (see "Reflex Hammer Technique" in Chapter 5). Upon asking the patient to lift up his great toe, there was no motion whatsoever; he could, however, lift (dorsiflex) his ankle a little, although this motion was very weak. I then proceeded to look at the proximal tibiofibular joint, as the common fibular nerve is located near the fibular head; I found this joint to be particularly stiff compared with the opposite side. I therefore decided to treat this specific joint by mobilization and soft-tissue work to the fibulares and tibialis anterior muscles. I was not sure what to expect from this treatment, but a few days later, the patient emailed me and thought he noticed a slight flicker of motion in his great toe. I continued with

this treatment to the head of the fibula and associated muscles; over the following weeks, the patient had some improvement, but the treatment was discontinued when until I felt we were not making any significant progress.

After my recommendation, the patient had a second MRI scan; this time the scan focused on his lower leg and specifically on the head of fibula and the anterior and lateral muscle compartments. The scan revealed something I had never seen before: there was an actual cyst approximately 20″ (8cm) long by 5″ (2cm), and the fluid was thought to be a "seepage" from the synovial fluid of the proximal tibiofibular joint. The scan also showed that the deep fibular nerve was encased within this cyst, which, to me, was the perfect explanation (in one respect) as to why this patient was presenting with drop foot. A few weeks later, the patient had surgery to remove the cyst, and as a result he has more movement in his great toe and ankle. However, several months after the surgery, there was still not total recovery of the nerve, and I believe the reason for this was that the initial compression damage to the deep fibular nerve caused by the cyst, and also the relatively long time it took to confirm the cyst's presence. I personally believe there will never be a full recovery, but on a positive note, the patient is a lot happier because a correct diagnosis has now been made and he has noticed some improvement to his ankle and foot.

Superior Gluteal Nerve

The *superior gluteal nerve* originates from L4, L5, and S1 and leaves the sacral plexus, passing through the greater sciatic foramen and over the piriformis, to innervate the following muscles:

- Tensor fasciae latae (TFL)
- Gluteus medius (Gmed)
- Gluteus minimus (Gmin)

Inferior Gluteal Nerve

The *inferior gluteal nerve* originates from L5, S1, and S2, and passes through the greater sciatic foramen and under the piriformis, to innervate the following muscle:

- Gluteus maximus (Gmax)

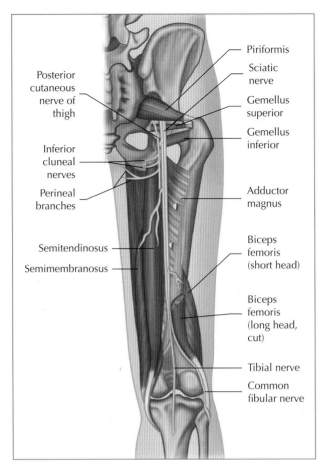

Figure 4.19: *Motor pathway of the posterior femoral cutaneous nerve.*

Posterior Femoral Cutaneous Nerve

The *posterior femoral cutaneous nerve* (Figure 4.19) exits the sacral plexus from S1–3 and travels through the greater sciatic foramen, passing below the piriformis. It provides the sensation to the skin over the posterior surface of the thigh and also to the perineum and buttocks.

Pudendal Nerve

The *pudendal nerve* (Figure 4.20) originates from the sacral plexus of S2–4 and passes through the lower part of the greater sciatic foramen, crossing over the sacrospinous ligament before entering the lesser sciatic foramen. It subsequently enters the *pudendal canal* to subdivide into the *inferior rectal nerve* and then into the superficial and deep *perineal nerve*.

The pudendal nerve supplies the sensation to the skin around the perineum and the anus, and also the genitalia of both sexes (the penis and scrotum in males, and the clitoris and labia majora in females). The motor supply is mainly to the external anal sphincter, external urethral sphincter, and the levator ani muscles of the pelvic floor.

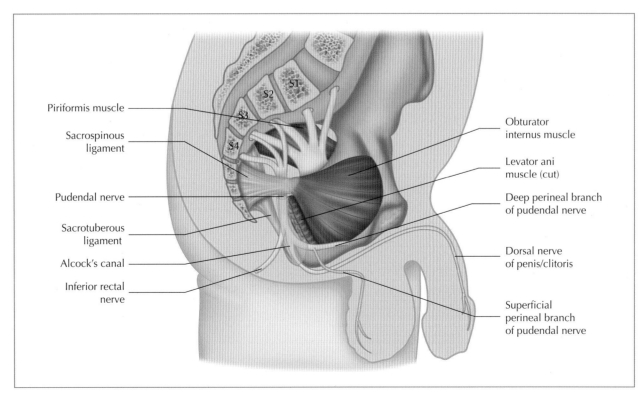

Figure 4.20: *Anatomy of the pudendal nerve and its divisions.*

CASE STUDY 4.3

A 75-year-old male came into the clinic with what he thought to be testicular symptoms, which had been bothering him for some time. He had seen the doctor, who did a testicular ultrasound; nothing of concern was found, so he was told to see a physical therapist. My initial thought process was that the sensory nerves (ilioinguinal/genitofemoral) that supplied the innervation to his groin region were involved, as they are in close proximity to the psoas major muscle. My initial treatment, therefore, was to focus on treating the psoas major through soft-tissue and lengthening techniques, and within two sessions his symptoms had settled down. I saw this man a few more times over the space of a year, but the last time I treated him, the effect on reducing his symptoms was minimal.

The patient now mentioned some other issues, however: problems with urination and increased frequency during the night, as well as the inability to maintain an erection. His doctor therefore palpated the prostate through the anal canal and found an irregularity with the organ. The doctor suggested blood tests to ascertain if the prostate was involved: this test is called a *prostate specific antigen* (PSA) test, which measures the amount of PSA in the blood. A PSA level of less than 4ng/ml is considered to be normal, but the value in this man's case was much higher: over 10ng/ml. The doctor said that the very high PSA level could be due to either an enlarged prostate (called *prostatic hyperplasia*), or sadly the possibility of prostate cancer.

The reason I mention Case Study 4.3 is because of the anatomical location of the prostate and the proximity to the associated nerves. You can see in Figure 4.21 that the nerve can be compressed by an increase in size of the prostate, potentially causing some of that patient's genital symptoms.

The patient was diagnosed with cancer; a few months later the prostate was removed and he made a full recovery.

Also supplied via the sacral plexus are the following muscles:

- Quadratus femoris (L4–5)
- Gemellus inferior (L5, S1, S2)
- Obturator internus and externus (L5, S1, S2)
- Gemellus superior (L5, S1, S2)
- Piriformis (L5, S1)

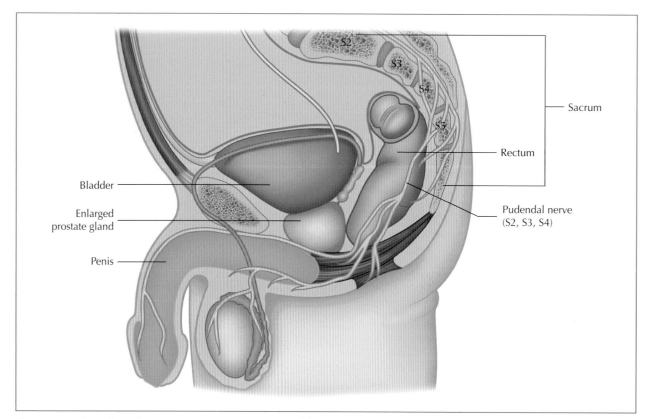

Figure 4.21: *An enlarged prostate causing compression of the associated nerves.*

5

Deep Tendon Reflexes

■ Reflex Responses

Most people have experienced their doctor tapping their knee with a rubber hammer. This is a very common procedure for testing the neurological system, as the simple motion of eliciting a reflex (or not, as the case may be) can detect pathology within the central or peripheral nervous systems.

The normal response to the practitioner tapping your knee is a *knee jerk*—this is a typical example of a deep tendon reflex (DTR), which, in this case, is an involuntary muscular response elicited by the patella or reflex hammer tapping the specific tendon. This response sends a signal via the afferent (sensory) nerve to the spinal cord and the message synapses at the inter neuron; the signal continues its journey via the efferent (motor) nerve back to the same muscle, subsequently causing a contraction and the jerk response, as shown in Figure 5.1.

The absence of a reflex response could be a clue that the spinal cord, nerve root, peripheral nerve, or the muscle

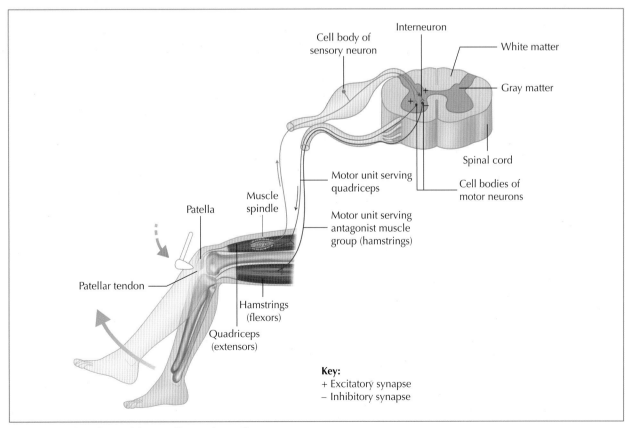

Figure 5.1: *Physiology of the patellar tendon reflex.*

has been damaged. When the reflex response is abnormal, this may be due to the disruption of the sensory (feeling) or motor (movement) nerves, or even both. To determine where the neural problem might be, the therapist tests reflexes in various parts of the body.

There are a variety of reflex hammers available to purchase and these are shown in Figure 5.2. My personal preference, however, is the larger plastic version called the *Queen Square*, which is the last one of the two plastic hammers on the far right of the five individual hammers shown in the figure. The triangular rubber hammer is the most popular and well known, especially in the US, and was actually the first known neurological reflex hammer; it was designed by John Madison Taylor in 1888 and is called the *Taylor* (or *Tomahawk*) *reflex hammer*.

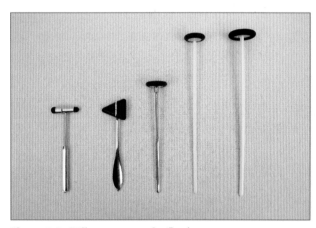

Figure 5.2: *Different types of reflex hammer.*

Many therapists, particularly in the UK, tend to buy the stainless-steel version because it typically contains a sharp testing point at one end and a light touch component at the other, as shown in Figure 5.3. These reflex hammers can be used to test the sensory areas of the related dermatomes.

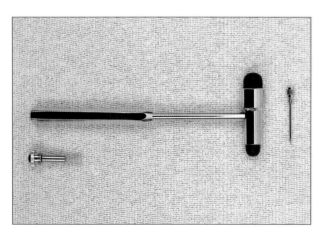

Figure 5.3: *Reflex hammer containing the extra sharp and light touch components.*

Reflex Hammer Technique

- Ensure that the patient is comfortable and relaxed, and that you can see the muscle being tested.
- Hold the end of the shaft of the hammer and strike the tendon (or you can tap your thumb placed over the tendon) of the specific muscle directly and look for muscle contraction.
- Repeat on the other side and compare the two.

A reflex can be classified as follows:

- *Hyperactive* (3+++)
- *Normal* (2++)
- *Sluggish* (1+)
- *Absent* (−)

■ Upper Limb Reflex Testing

C5 Reflex Test—Biceps

- Ask the patient to relax their arm and hold their elbow between your thumb and remaining fingers.
- Instruct them to resist elbow flexion, so that you can feel the contraction of the biceps tendon.
- With your thumb placed directly over the biceps tendon, elicit the biceps reflex by tapping the hammer gently on your thumb (Figure 5.4).

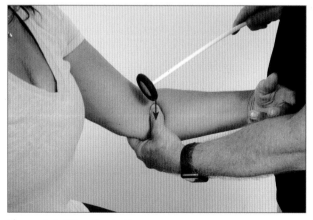

Figure 5.4: *C5 reflex testing.*

The C5 biceps reflex is conducted through the musculo-skeletal nerve of the brachial plexus, as shown in Figure 5.5.

C6 Reflex Test—Brachioradialis

- Ask the patient to relax their arm and gently grasp their wrist.

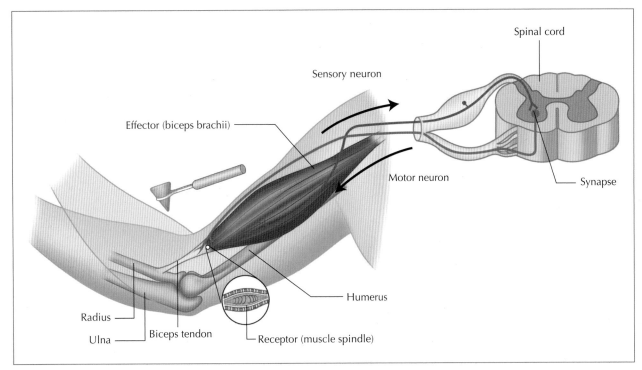

Figure 5.5: *C5 reflex testing through the musculocutaneous nerve.*

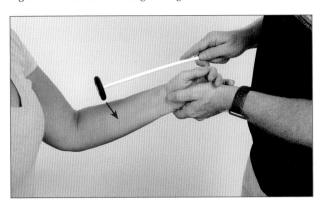

Figure 5.6: *C6 reflex testing.*

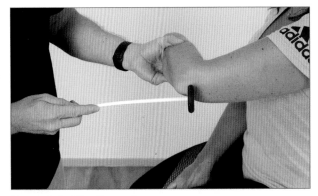

Figure 5.7: *C7 reflex testing.*

- Instruct them to elbow flex, so that you can see the contraction of the brachioradialis muscle.
- Elicit the brachioradialis reflex by tapping gently over the brachioradialis tendon just above the wrist (or even over the muscle belly, as this also works) (Figure 5.6).

The C6 brachioradialis reflex is conducted through the radial nerve.

C7 Reflex Test—Triceps

- Hold the patient's relaxed arm across their lower chest/upper abdomen with one of your hands.
- Elicit the triceps reflex by tapping over the triceps tendon just above and behind their olecranon (triceps insertion point located on the ulna) of the elbow (Figure 5.7).

The C7 triceps reflex is conducted through the radial nerve.

Note: If a particular reflex is difficult to elicit, try the same technique with a "reinforcement"—ask the patient to clench their teeth or interlock their fingers and try to pull their fingers apart, while you try again to elicit the reflex.

Reflex testing upper limb

■ Lower Limb Reflex Testing

L3 Reflex Test—Adductors

- With the patient's leg relaxed, locate their adductor longus muscle and ask them to resist adduction, so that you can feel the contraction of the tendon.
- Next, place two fingers onto the tendon and apply pressure, as this will change the tension within the tissue.
- Elicit the adductor reflex by tapping the hammer gently on your fingers (Figure 5.8).

The L3 adductor reflex is conducted through the obturator nerve.

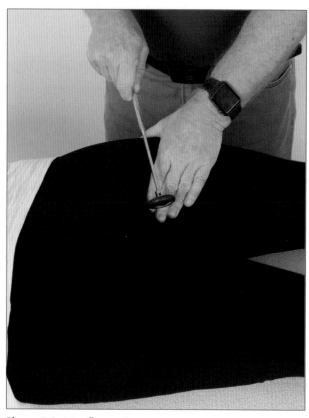

Figure 5.8: *L3 reflex testing.*

L4 Reflex Test—Patellar Tendon

- Ask the patient to relax their leg, and gently grasp it and take it into flexion of around 20 degrees.
- Elicit the patellar tendon reflex by tapping gently over the patellar tendon, as shown in Figure 5.9 (in this case, you do not need to put your thumb on the tendon).

The L4 patellar tendon reflex is conducted through the femoral nerve.

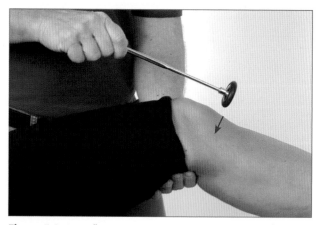

Figure 5.9: *L4 reflex testing.*

L5 Reflex Test—Medial Hamstring Tendon

The medial hamstring tendon has been demonstrated by Esene et al. (2012) to be an effective way to test the L5 reflex, although not many therapists are aware of this unique reflex.

- Ask the patient to assume a prone position and to relax their leg.
- Next, gently grasp the leg and take the knee into flexion of around 30 degrees.
- Elicit the L5 reflex by tapping gently on your thumb placed over the medial hamstring tendon of either the semitendinosus or the semimembranosus, as shown in Figure 5.10.

The L5 medial hamstring reflex is conducted through the tibial nerve (a component of the sciatic nerve).

S1 Reflex Testing—Achilles

- Hold the patient's relaxed leg and slowly bend their knee and take their leg into abduction and external rotation.
- Apply dorsiflexion to the ankle to stretch the tendon.
- Elicit the Achilles reflex by tapping directly over the Achilles tendon just above the heel bone (Figure 5.11).

The S1 Achilles reflex is conducted through the tibial nerve (a component of the sciatic nerve).

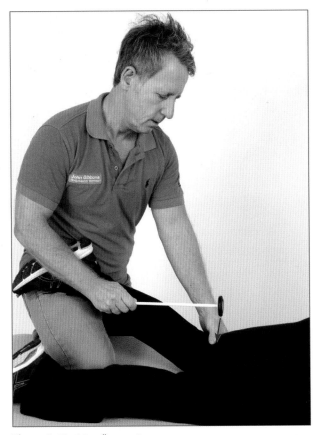

Figure 5.10: *L5 reflex testing.*

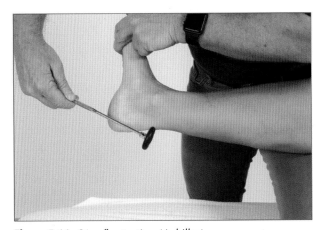

Figure 5.11: *S1 reflex testing (Achilles).*

S1 Reflex Test—Plantar Surface of Foot

This is an alternative to the above Achilles test and is classified as an *S1 reflex test*.

- With the patient's leg relaxed, slowly apply dorsiflexion to the ankle with two fingers over the plantar surface of the foot.

- Elicit the plantar reflex by tapping over the ball of the foot just adjacent to your fingers (Figure 5.12).

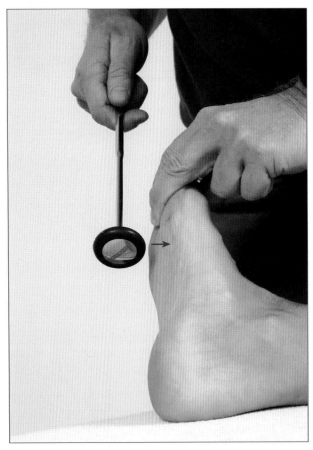

Figure 5.12: *S1 reflex testing (plantar).*

The S1 plantar reflex is conducted through the plantar nerve, which is a continuation of the tibial nerve (a component of the sciatic nerve).

S3–4 Reflex Test—External Anal Sphincter

This relatively invasive test will ascertain the ability of the innervation of the pudendal nerve (S2–4); the procedure should cause a contracture of the anal sphincter, also known as an *anal wink*. Naturally, this test is only performed when the practitioner considers it of importance to the assessment process.

Reflex testing—lower limb

- Lightly contact the patient's anus with a piece of cotton wool, and look for a response.
- This light touch should induce a reflex contracture of the anal sphincter muscles, as shown in Figure 5.13.

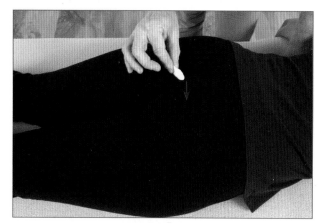

Figure 5.13: *Light touching of the anus induces a contraction of the anal sphincter.*

Babinski Reflex Test—Plantar Surface of Foot

The Babinski reflex test, named after the neurologist Joseph Babinski, is a specific neurological test that can detect pathology within the central nervous system of either the brain or the spinal cord. However, in the newborn baby (until 12–24 months of age), this test shows positive because at this young age, the corticospinal tracts that run from the brain to the spinal cord are not fully myelinated. As the baby develops control over their neurological system, the Babinski response disappears.

- Expose the skin of the foot of the patient and run a blunt object up and along the lateral side of the plantar surface of the foot, starting at the heel area and finishing toward the toes. The end of a metal reflex hammer is ideal for this, but be careful because sometimes it can be sharp.
- There are typically one of three responses elicited:
  - A *normal response* (or the Babinski sign is absent) is where the toes curl down and inward, as shown in Figure 5.14(a).
  - A *no response* is where there is no motion elicited in the foot.
  - A *positive response* (or the Babinski sign is present) is where you will notice the hallux extending (dorsiflexion) and the toes spanning out, as shown in Figure 5.14(b).

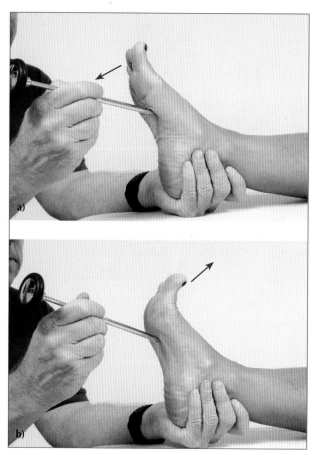

Figure 5.14: *Babinski reflex testing: (a) normal response; (b) positive response.*

If you observe the third response, where the hallux dorsiflexes and the other toes span out, then you know that there is pathology located within the CNS (Figure 5.14(b)), and further investigation is warranted. If the Babinski reflex occurs on one side of the foot and not on the other, then this indicates pathology in one side of the brain. Typically, these positive Babinski tests necessitate further investigation, which might include a computed tomography (CT) scan of the brain, an MRI of the spinal cord, and/or a lumbar puncture to test the cerebrospinal fluid.

Babinski reflex test

■ Examples of Interpretations of Findings

Upper Motor Neuron Lesion

An upper motor neuron (UMN) lesion typically produces *hyperreflexia* (increased reflex), and the Babinski reflex is one of the main clinical tests. The response is normally positive (up-pointing toes), and there will also be hypertonicity (increased muscle tone) and spasticity, which is usually felt when the patient's limb is passively moved quickly, as a resistance to the motion can then be detected. There is generally a clonus present, which is where the stretch reflex is so strong that the muscle is seen to contract 4–7 times. This is reminiscent of an oscillatory type of motion and can usually be elicited from the ankle when the joint is suddenly stretched into dorsiflexion.

Lower Motor Neuron Lesion

A lower motor neuron (LMN) lesion typically produces *hyporeflexia* (diminished or absent response to reflex testing), hypotonicity (reduced muscle tone), fasciculation (involuntary muscle twitching) and fibrillation (you may possibly feel this reaction of the muscle but not actually see the contraction as an EMG is required for its detection), and weakness with muscle atrophy (muscle wastage).

The differences between the upper and lower motor neuron lesions are listed in Table 5.1.

Table 5.1: Differences between upper and lower motor neuron lesions.

UMN lesion symptoms	LMN lesion symptoms
Hyperreflexia	Hyporeflexia
Hypertonicity	Hypotonicity
Spasticity	Flaccid paralysis
Babinski reflex positive	Babinski reflex negative
Clonus present	Fasciculation and fibrillation

An isolated loss of a reflex can point to a radiculopathy affecting that specific spinal segment; for example, there may be a loss of biceps reflex if there is a C4–5 disc prolapse that is contacting the exiting nerve root of C5.

■ Quick Reference Table of Specific Reflexes

Table 5.2: Specific reflexes for the upper and lower limbs.

Area tested for reflex	Corresponding spinal level
Biceps tendon	C5
Brachioradialis (forearm)	C6
Triceps (elbow)	C7
Adductors	L3
Patellar tendon	L4
Medial hamstrings	L5
Achilles tendon	S1
Plantar (foot)	S1
External anal sphincter	S3/S4
Babinski (plantar)	Upper motor neuron (CNS)

I cannot overemphasize the importance of reflex testing. If you only learn one thing from this book, then please become competent in the use of the reflex hammer, because it can really be a great help in ascertaining correct diagnoses of your patients.

The next section presents a few case studies involving real people who have visited the clinic in Oxford, and you will see shortly just how important reflex testing was in these cases.

■ Case Studies

CASE STUDY 5.1

A 24-year-old male came to see me with what he described as a weak left leg. He was very active and enjoyed martial arts. He mentioned that his right leg was strong when he kicked, but when he tried to kick with his left leg, there was something obviously wrong; no matter what he tried, he felt that the signals from his brain were not getting through to his leg (that is how he described it in his own words). The patient also mentioned some lower thoracic pain. He had attended over twenty sessions with a chiropractor and physical therapists for the last few months, but still felt the discomfort of the thoracic pain; more importantly, there had been no change in his leg symptoms.

After my initial consultation, the *first* thing I decided to do in terms of the examination was to use my patella (reflex) hammer and check his reflexes. I found the upper limb of C5, C6, and C7 to be normal (2++); however, the lower limb reflexes of L4 and S1 were noticeably different, as I found them to be very brisk (3+++). I carried out the Babinski reflex on both of his feet and found the hallux and toes to go up (extension) instead of coming down (flexion), which is a *positive* finding for a lesion within the upper motor neurons of the CNS.

When I teach my students, I say to them that we are all like detectives, but what I would more aptly call *therapy detectives*. The patient gives us information and we then have to try to work out what might be going on. It is not as easy as it sounds, but over time and with experience, we eventually become more knowledgeable, as everything in life is a learning curve. Regarding this patient, and to recap a little on my basic findings, the upper reflexes of C5, C6, and C7 were normal when tested. I considered that the brain and spinal cord (CNS) was working normally from the levels C7 and above, but something was not quite right from the levels L4 to C7, because the reflexes were brisk and the Babinski response was positive.

Let me discuss that concept for a moment, as some readers might be a little confused about what it is I am trying to explain. If all the reflexes were brisk (3+++) and the Babinski reflex positive, this would point to an *upper motor neuron* (UMN) *lesion*, so the problem would be isolated within the brain or spinal cord (CNS). However, the upper reflexes tested normal (2++), so I knew the problem had to be *below* the C7 level and *above* the L4 level, because the lower reflexes were brisk and the Babinski reflex was positive. Hopefully that makes a little more sense. I therefore reasoned that there was something within the actual spinal cord between L4 and C7 that was not quite right because of the altered reflexes.

The patient mentioned some pain in his lower thoracic spine, so I concluded that there must be an issue with his spinal cord at those specific levels of the thoracic spine. I knew there must be some form of pathology located within the upper motor neuron (central nervous system), because the reflexes were brisk and the Babinski reflex was positive. I spoke to his doctor, who arranged an immediate MRI scan to his cervical, thoracic, and lumbar spines; the diagnosis was a *neurofibroma* located between the levels of T9–11.

As a result of the diagnosis, the patient subsequently had spinal surgery to remove the tumor, and a few months later he came back to see me. I was pleased to find that the left leg and reflexes were normal and that he no longer had pain in his thoracic spine.

Paraplegia

From a negative perspective, if the patient in Case Study 5.1 had not gone through surgery and the condition had continued to progress, there would have been the possibility of him developing a condition called *paraplegia*. This is an impairment of the motor or sensory nervous systems, affecting the lower extremities (both legs), with the cause being located in either the thoracic or the lumbar spine. The chances of a full recovery might then have been limited. If the spinal lesion had been higher up and located in the cervical spine, his upper extremities as well as his lower extremities might have been affected, a condition called *quadriplegia*, also known as *tetraplegia*.

CASE STUDY 5.2

A 45-year-old female sent me an email describing a hip and groin problem that had been present for some time, and asked if could I have a look at her to see if I could help. She came to see me, and during the consultation I believed that there was a little more going on than just the matter of her hip joint. She kept on saying things to me that did not quite add up: for example, she started to notice that there was something wrong with one of her eyes, and she also had an awareness of weakness issues in certain parts of her body, even though this was rather vague in her description.

I nevertheless assessed her hip joint, as that was the main reason for coming to see me, and I did say that I felt she might have a labral (cartilage) issue within the hip joint that would require further investigation. I then asked my patient if I could assess her neurological system through the use of the patella hammer, to which she replied, "Yes, of course." I found all of her reflexes to be rather brisk (3+++) and the Babinski reflex (located on the plantar surface of the foot) to be positive, with the toes responding in an upward extending manner rather than in a downward motion (flexion). I discussed these findings with my patient and inquired if there were any neurological issues in her family; her reply was "No."

I wrote a letter to her doctor, and a few weeks later she was diagnosed with multiple sclerosis (MS) through an

MRI scan of her brain. She phoned me after her diagnosis, thanking me for seeing her and referring her to the doctor, and surprisingly asked me what she could do about her hip. I said that, given the circumstances of her MS diagnosis, the hip issue was relatively inconsequential in the grand scheme of things, and that she should focus on making the most out of her life, because you never know what this disease has in store for you in the long term.

Multiple Sclerosis

Multiple sclerosis (MS) is an autoimmune disorder and, for some unknown reason, the body attacks itself; in particular, the condition causes a demyelination of the myelin insulating layer in the brain or spinal cord. Sadly, there is no underlying cause of this upper motor neuron disease and no cure, but certain types of medication might help.

Some typical symptoms of MS experienced by a patient are:

- Visual disturbances (one of the most common symptoms)
- Numbness and tingling of the face, arms, fingers, and legs
- Difficulty in walking and in controlling gait
- Balance issues and dizziness
- Cognitive problems
- Issues with control of the bladder and bowel
- Pain and muscle spasms with spasticity
- Speech and swallowing difficulties
- Depression
- Anxiety
- Fatigue and weakness

CASE STUDY 5.3

A 51-year-old female came to see me with what she described as an ongoing neck problem; she also mentioned some weakness in one of her hands. This problem had been ongoing for some time and seemed to be getting progressively worse, so she asked me if I could have a look at her to see if I could help.

During the consultation, I considered that there was a little more going on than just a simple cervical facet or disc problem that was referring to her hand. She maintained that she was having difficulty holding certain objects in her left hand and that this hand felt clumsy

compared with the right, and insisted that she noticed a slight tremor was developing in her left hand as well. There was also some mention of her losing her balance from time to time, and of her usual walking pattern not seeming the same as it used to be.

When I was training as an osteopath, one of the tutors kept emphasizing the importance of using a reflex hammer with every patient who visits the clinic; I therefore decided that this would be my goal as well, i.e., to use some form of neurological testing with the majority of my patients.

When I tested this patient with the reflex hammer, I found all of her reflexes to be very brisk, with a grade of 3+++, which I classified as *hyperreflexia*. I then decided to perform the Babinski reflex on her foot and found this to be normal. Next, I asked her to touch her index finger, then middle, ring, and little fingers, with her thumb, and to try to repeat this exercise quickly. Performing this simple task was no problem with her right hand, but proved difficult with her left hand. She said she was trying to send the information to her hand, but for some reason the messages did not seem to be getting through.

I referred this patient to her medical doctor, and a diagnosis of early stage Parkinson's disease was pronounced.

Parkinson's Disease

Parkinson's disease (PD) is a consequence of another upper motor neuron lesion and typically occurs between 50 and 65 years of age. The disease has been proven to be caused mainly by the death of dopamine-producing cells (chemical messengers known as *neurotransmitters*) located within the substantia nigra (Latin for "black substance," as it looks like a darkened streak within the brain tissue). The *substantia nigra* is located within the brain where the spinal cord meets the mid-brain and is a natural part of the system called the *basal ganglia*, responsible for turning our thoughts about movements into action, as the basal ganglia controls voluntary motor movements. The substantia nigra is the main regulator and needs a constant supply of dopamine to communicate with the basal ganglia; without this chemical, altered movement symptoms will start to appear. An imbalance of the signals within the basal ganglia can cause the resting hand tremor that is typically seen with PD.

PD is also partly caused by the death of ACh-producing cells, another chemical messenger known as a *neurotransmitter*. The actual cause of the death of these cells is unknown, but what is known is that approximately 80% of the dopamine-producing cells have already died before any symptoms of the disease appear. The loss of these cells in the basal ganglia now affects the motor areas of the cerebral cortex, subsequently decreasing voluntary movements.

The progression of PD has been classified into five stages, which vary from mild to severe, and some of the signs and symptoms of the disease are:

- Difficulty in standing up from a sitting position
- Shuffling of the feet during the gait cycle, with absent arm swing
- Stooped posture
- Rigidity—upper limb "cog-wheel" rigidity and lower limb "lead-pipe" rigidity
- Resting tremor, known as a *pill rolling tremor*
- Loss of facial expression—mask-like facial features
- Slurring of speech
- Tendency to develop dementia later

Conclusion

Hopefully, Case Studies 5.1–5.3 demonstrate the importance of the use of the reflex hammer, as well as a thorough case history. Honestly, with my hand on my heart, if I had not used the hammer, I might not have considered the problems in these cases to be related to neurological conditions (apart from Parkinson's).

If you think about Case Study 5.1, if I had not tested the reflexes, I would have simply carried on treating the patient's thoracic spine, and he would no doubt have progressively gotten worse. As regards Case Study 5.2, again if I had not tested that patient's reflexes, I would have focused on treating just the hip joint, rather than considering anything else, as that is what she came to see me for in the first place.

The overall prognosis for the patient in Case Study 5.1 improved dramatically, and he made a full recovery after the surgery. In Case Study 5.2, however, the eventual prognosis of MS is not so clear. For the third patient, with a diagnosis of Parkinson's, the Babinski reflex tends to be normal with this disease, even though the condition is located within the brain. That patient was prescribed L-dopa medication, which is currently working, as it helps increase the dopamine concentration and can cross the blood-brain barrier (dopamine itself cannot directly cross this barrier). Unfortunately, this drug typically has side effects and is not effective as a cure for the disease, since the condition is progressive and the medication will only work for a certain length of time.

Remember, your role as a physical therapist is to be able to help and provide reassurance to your patients, no matter what the diagnosis and prognosis turn out to be.

Reflex testing—upper & lower limb

6

Sensory Testing—Dermatomes and Cutaneous Nerves

■ Examination of the Sensory System (Dermatome)

What is a Dermatome?

A *dermatome* is a specific area of skin located on the body that is innervated by a single nerve root (Figure 6.1).

The difficulty with looking at maps of dermatomes is that there is a certain amount of diversity in terms of the information they provide. What I mean by this is that there is no real consistency between the dermatome maps that can be found on the internet, for example. If you look at, say, four or five maps on different websites (and the same goes for neurological books), they will all have slight variations. In consequence, one might say, it is actually pretty confusing for the beginner who is trying to learn about this subject. I totally agree with this, but hopefully it is not too much of an issue, because you have to remember we are all individuals and unique in our own DNA, so our own personal dermatome map might be slightly different from somebody else's!

If you have experienced symptoms such as numbness, tingling, burning sensations, skin crawling, itching, and pain, you can describe them as sharp, shooting, or stabbing, or simply as constant and ongoing. In reality, all of these symptoms are different types of neurological sensation, and they may be felt in any areas of the upper and lower limbs as well as in the extremities, such as the hands and feet. Sometimes these symptoms radiate from one area into another; sciatica is a good example of pain that can radiate into the lower extremity.

What is a Cutaneous Nerve?

Cutaneous nerve innervation is related to just the sensory area of the *skin*, and a specific *cutaneous nerve* supplies this area. If you look at Figure 6.2 you will see a map of the cutaneous nerves of the body, all of which are sensory nerves. A dermatome, on the other hand, is similar, but the area of innervation is related to only a single spinal nerve root.

It is not always easy to distinguish between pain or altered sensations from a spinal nerve root or from a cutaneous innervation, so let's look at some examples. For the first example, suppose you have sustained trauma to the cervical spine and there is a confirmed C4/5 disc bulge on an MRI scan. There is a possibility of experiencing referred sensations, such as pain, numbness, and tingling, along the C5 spinal nerve root (dermatome) because of the compression of the exiting C5 nerve root. This is called *radiculopathy*, hence the referral to the specific dermatome area.

As a second example, let's say you have had knee surgery. In this case, you might lose some sensation in the knee area because the surgeon has cut the superficial cutaneous nerve.

A third example relates to a friend of mine who damaged his radial nerve near his elbow, and subsequently lost some of the feeling in his forearm and the web space of his thumb. The altered sensations he perceived were not due to a cervical disc problem that followed a C6 dermatome pattern, but rather to damage to a cutaneous (sensory) part of the radial nerve.

We have all knocked our elbow at some point and felt a sharp or tingling sensation in the tip of our little finger. This uncomfortable sensation occurs because we contacted the ulnar nerve, and the microdamage caused a response to be sent to the area this nerve supplies (i.e., the little finger). Thus, the source of the referral cannot

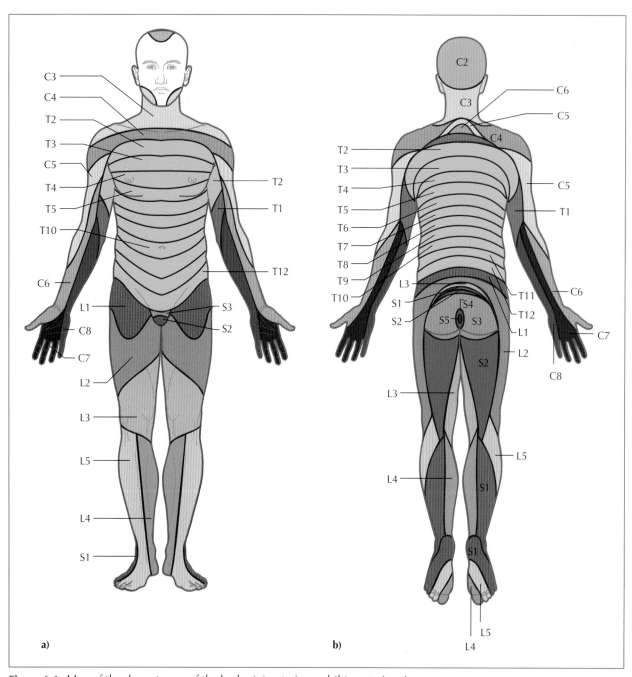

Figure 6.1: *Map of the dermatomes of the body: (a) anterior and (b) posterior views.*

in reality be along a dermatome pathway that has been referred from a spinal nerve root (C8). This should clarify the differences between dermatomes and cutaneous nerve innervations.

Figure 6.3 presents a comparison of the dermatomes and cutaneous nerve supplies of the anterior and posterior regions of the body.

Paresthesia

Paresthesia is generally the term used to describe some of the symptoms listed above, and typically the words that patients might use are "prickling or burning sensations," usually felt in the arms, hands, legs, and feet. No doubt you have all experienced "pins and needles," especially after having slept with your arm in an awkward position, or sometimes if you happened to just contact your elbow on the inside, producing a sudden electric-shock type of feeling that usually extends to your little finger, as you have irritated the ulnar nerve. The good thing about the above symptoms is that they are often only temporary, as they are typically painless as well as harmless, and they should disappear fairly quickly. However, for some people with underlying neurological conditions, this is not the case, and the paresthesia may be caused by actual nerve damage, called *neuropathy*.

Anesthesia

Anesthesia is a loss of sensation, while *hypoesthesia* is a decrease in sensation. Numbness is the most common symptom that patients might report: "I cannot seem to feel that area of my body." It could simply be the site of knee surgery, and one of the superficial cutaneous nerves has been cut during the procedure, so the patient is unable to feel a certain part of their skin over the knee. Sometimes pregnancy can cause a compression of the lateral femoral cutaneous nerve, since this is located near to the anterior superior iliac spine (ASIS) as the nerve passes under or through the inguinal ligament; the person might remark that they "cannot feel the outside part of the thigh," as it feels numb when they rub it.

Hyperesthesia

Hyperesthesia is an abnormal increase in sensitivity of any of your senses (sight, sound, touch, and smell); if it relates to the skin and to increased touch sensation, it is called *tactile hyperesthesia*. Tactile hyperesthesia can cause the patient to suffer severe pain when their nerves are triggered; for example, this can occur if the nerves are partially or completely impaired by increased blood sugars, as this can cause peripheral neuropathy (diabetes). Hyperesthesia can also be related to increased sensitivity to the food we eat and to the sounds we hear (*auditory hyperesthesia*); increased sensitivity can also be caused by a vitamin B12 deficiency, but supplementation will normally eliminate the problem.

■ Dermatomes

Nerves originate from the spinal cord and divide into sensory and motor nerves. The sensory nerves provide sensation to specific areas of the skin; these nerves are known as *dermatomes*. The dermatome patterns have the appearance of a map on the body. The therapist may use a piece of cotton wool, a pin, or even a paperclip to test symmetrical feelings in the arms and legs. Abnormal responses by the patient when tested may be indicative of a specific nerve root problem.

Because of the thousands of nerve endings located within the skin, each of us should be able to ascertain the difference between four specific sensations detected by the skin, namely:

- Hot
- Cold
- Pain
- Pressure

There are actually 30 numbered dermatomes and these are related to the spinal levels that they originate from. There is no C1 dermatome, as this level has no sensory root, so the dermatomes start from C2 and finish at S5, as seen in Tables 6.2–6.4. We tend to separate the dermatomes into upper limb and lower limb, as these are the areas most commonly tested by the practitioner. However, there are 12 thoracic dermatomes that deserve a mention as well.

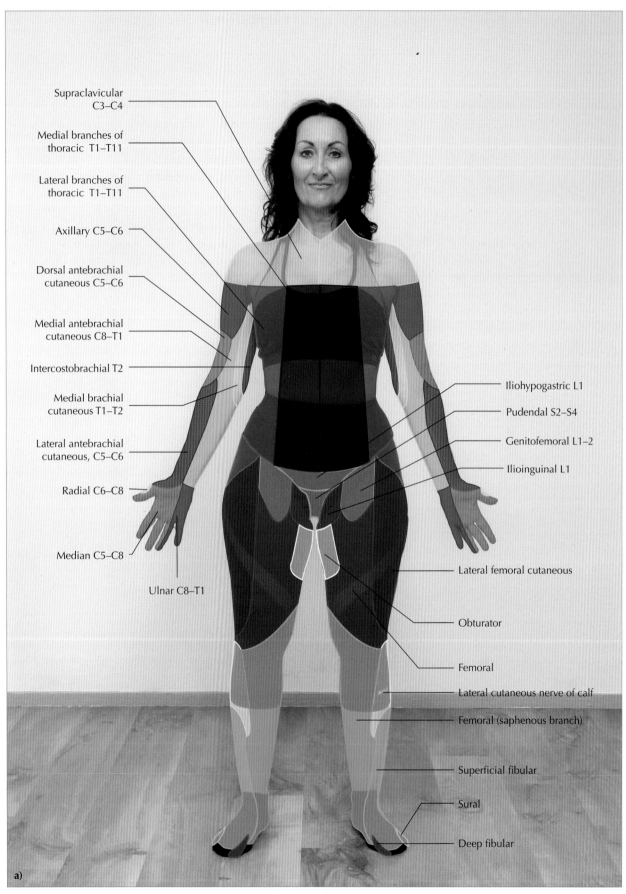

Supraclavicular
C3–C4

Medial branches of
thoracic T1–T11

Lateral branches of
thoracic T1–T11

Axillary C5–C6

Dorsal antebrachial
cutaneous C5–C6

Medial antebrachial
cutaneous C8–T1

Intercostobrachial T2

Medial brachial
cutaneous T1–T2

Lateral antebrachial
cutaneous, C5–C6

Radial C6–C8

Median C5–C8

Ulnar C8–T1

Iliohypogastric L1

Pudendal S2–S4

Genitofemoral L1–2

Ilioinguinal L1

Lateral femoral cutaneous

Obturator

Femoral

Lateral cutaneous nerve of calf

Femoral (saphenous branch)

Superficial fibular

Sural

Deep fibular

a)

Figure 6.2a: *Map of the cutaneous nerves of the body (anterior view).*

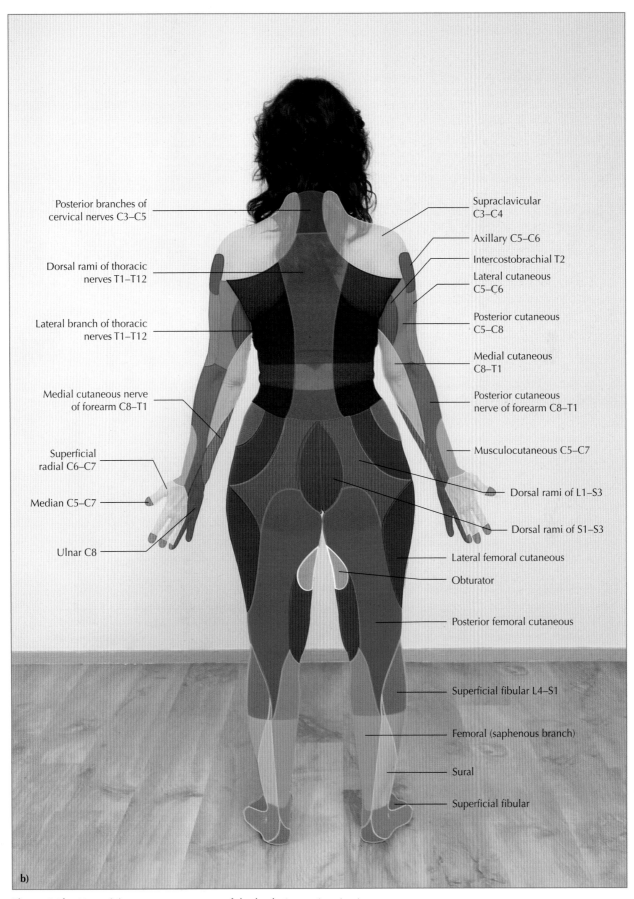

Posterior branches of
cervical nerves C3–C5

Dorsal rami of thoracic
nerves T1–T12

Lateral branch of thoracic
nerves T1–T12

Medial cutaneous nerve
of forearm C8–T1

Superficial
radial C6–C7

Median C5–C7

Ulnar C8

Supraclavicular
C3–C4

Axillary C5–C6

Intercostobrachial T2

Lateral cutaneous
C5–C6

Posterior cutaneous
C5–C8

Medial cutaneous
C8–T1

Posterior cutaneous
nerve of forearm C8–T1

Musculocutaneous C5–C7

Dorsal rami of L1–S3

Dorsal rami of S1–S3

Lateral femoral cutaneous

Obturator

Posterior femoral cutaneous

Superficial fibular L4–S1

Femoral (saphenous branch)

Sural

Superficial fibular

b)

Figure 6.2b: *Map of the cutaneous nerves of the body (posterior view).*

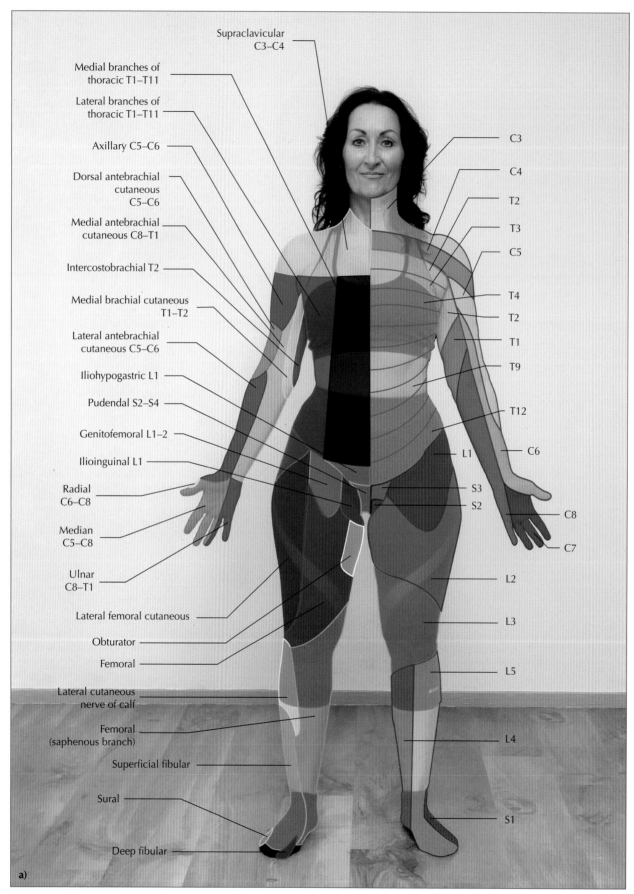

Supraclavicular
C3–C4

Medial branches of
thoracic T1–T11

Lateral branches of
thoracic T1–T11

Axillary C5–C6

Dorsal antebrachial
cutaneous
C5–C6

Medial antebrachial
cutaneous C8–T1

Intercostobrachial T2

Medial brachial cutaneous
T1–T2

Lateral antebrachial
cutaneous C5–C6

Iliohypogastric L1

Pudendal S2–S4

Genitofemoral L1–2

Ilioinguinal L1

Radial
C6–C8

Median
C5–C8

Ulnar
C8–T1

Lateral femoral cutaneous

Obturator

Femoral

Lateral cutaneous
nerve of calf

Femoral
(saphenous branch)

Superficial fibular

Sural

Deep fibular

C3

C4

T2

T3

C5

T4

T2

T1

T9

T12

L1

C6

S3

S2

C8

C7

L2

L3

L5

L4

S1

a)

Figure 6.3a: *Comparison of a map of the dermatomes and the cutaneous nerves of the body (anterior view).*

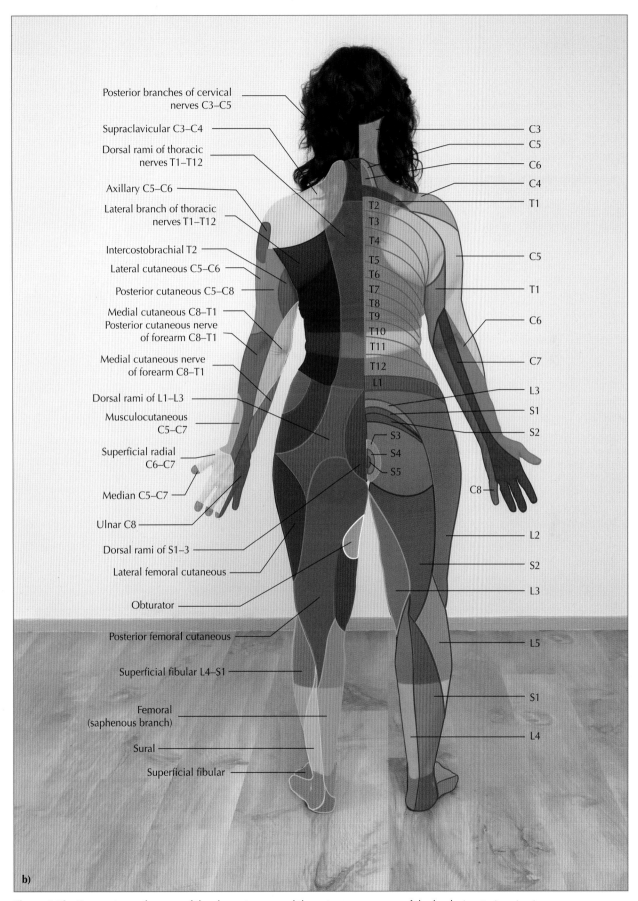

Posterior branches of cervical nerves C3–C5

Supraclavicular C3–C4

Dorsal rami of thoracic nerves T1–T12

Axillary C5–C6

Lateral branch of thoracic nerves T1–T12

Intercostobrachial T2

Lateral cutaneous C5–C6

Posterior cutaneous C5–C8

Medial cutaneous C8–T1
Posterior cutaneous nerve of forearm C8–T1

Medial cutaneous nerve of forearm C8–T1

Dorsal rami of L1–L3

Musculocutaneous C5–C7

Superficial radial C6–C7

Median C5–C7

Ulnar C8

Dorsal rami of S1–3

Lateral femoral cutaneous

Obturator

Posterior femoral cutaneous

Superficial fibular L4–S1

Femoral (saphenous branch)

Sural

Superficial fibular

C3
C5
C6
C4
T1
T2
T3
T4
T5
T6
T7
T8
T9
T10
T11
T12
L1
C5
T1
C6
C7
L3
S1
S2
S3
S4
S5
C8
L2
S2
L3
L5
S1
L4

b)

Figure 6.3b: *Comparison of a map of the dermatomes and the cutaneous nerves of the body (posterior view).*

Table 6.1: A dermatome versus a cutaneous nerve.

Dermatome	Cutaneous nerve
A *dermatome* is a sensory region located on the body that is supplied by a single spinal nerve root.	*Cutaneous innervation* is a localized sensory region of the skin that is innervated by a specific cutaneous nerve.

Table 6.2: Map of the dermatomes of the upper body.

Dermatome location—upper body	Spinal level
Occipital protuberance and posterior neck	C2
Anterior neck and supraclavicular fossa	C3
Supraclavicular fossa and acromioclavicular joint	C4
Infraclavicular area and across upper limb to above elbow	C5
Lateral forearm and thumb	C6
Middle finger	C7
Little finger	C8
Medial forearm	T1

Table 6.3: Map of the dermatomes of the thoracic spine.

Dermatome location—thoracic spine	Spinal level
Medial forearm	T1
Medial upper arm and axilla	T2
Superior to nipple line	T3
Level of nipple line	T4
Superior to xiphoid process	T5
Level of xiphoid process	T6
Inferior to xiphoid process	T7
Halfway between xiphoid process and umbilicus	T8
Superior to umbilicus	T9
Level of umbilicus	T10
Inferior to umbilicus	T11
Suprapubic area, level with iliac crest	T12

■ Sensory Tests

To accurately assess the neurological sensory components, especially of the dermatomes, we can use some simple pieces of equipment (Figure 6.4), such as cotton wool, a Neurotip, even a hatpin, or a tuning fork, or we could simply (subject to consent) use our fingers and touch our patients gently or with applied pressure. When I see my patients, I personally do not include all of the following sensory tests discussed in this section; however, I do use some of them in my assessment of the neurological

Table 6.4: Map of the dermatomes of the lower body.

Dermatome location—lower body	Spinal level
Below inguinal ligament, groin	L1
Upper thigh	L2
Anterior thigh to knee	L3
Medial aspect of lower leg and medial malleolus	L4
Lateral aspect of lower leg, dorsum of foot and toes 1–4	L5
Lateral aspect of foot and little toe, lateral malleolus, heel, and majority of sole of foot	S1
Posterior aspect of thigh and popliteal fossa	S2
Concentric rings around anus (we sit on S3), area of ischial tuberosity	S3
Skin over perianal area and genitals	S4
Skin next to anus as well as perianal area	S5

Note: I mentioned the lack of map consistency earlier, and I consider it an interesting peculiarity in one respect that some dermatome maps show the L5 dermatome covering the great toe (hallux), while others show the L4 dermatome covering that particular area. Just bear in mind, therefore, that variations do exist, and so it is difficult to say which one is actually correct.

system. The basic idea of these tests is to ascertain if the patient actually has a neurological issue, as some individuals might not be aware of contact to their skin through the use of an external source.

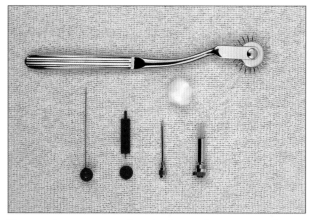

Figure 6.4: *Instruments that can be used to ascertain the function of the sensory nervous system (dermatomes).*

The primary role of the sensory nervous system is to process specific sensations that provide ongoing sensory feedback from the outside world (via the skin) to the CNS. As long as there are no underlying neurological conditions present, then each of us should be able to distinguish the following five different types of sensation:

- Light touch
- Sharpness/bluntness (pressure)

- Temperature (hot and cold)
- Vibration
- Joint position sense (JPS—proprioception)

The reason why we might use five tests instead of one is because there are several different pathways back to the CNS which carry the sensory information; for example, large myelinated nerve fibers carry information from vibration and joint position sensations, and these fibers are located directly within the *posterior columns* of the spinal cord. The sensations from pain and temperature, however, return to the CNS via smaller unmyelinated nerve fibers; these travel back through the *spinothalamic tracts* within the spinal cord. Light touch is a combination of both of these transport systems.

The point of mentioning the different sensory pathways is that if you were to lose one or two types of sensation, the other types of sensation could remain intact. For example, in multiple sclerosis, which is a demyelination of the CNS, the most common sensory deficit relates to vibration. This is most noticeable in the feet and is caused by a demyelination of the posterior columns. The transport of sensory information derived from pain or temperature (unmyelinated nerve fibers), however, would not be affected.

Light Touch

For testing light touch, a finger, a piece of cotton wool, or a piece of tissue paper is used. It is important to touch and not to stroke (which would otherwise be a moving sensation).

- Demonstrate first by contacting the patient with a light touch, so that they understand the procedure and say the word "yes" when they feel the contact.
- Next, ask the patient to close their eyes, and to tell you when they feel you touching them by saying "yes."
- All the testing should be done to specific dermatomes and compared bilaterally.
- Keep the timing of each touch irregular in order to avoid anticipation by the patient; for example, test C5 on the right arm, then C7 on the left arm, then C6 on the right arm, etc.
- Note any areas of reduced or increased sensation.

Figure 6.5(a) and (b) show light touch being applied by a piece of cotton wool to the specific dermatomes of the upper limb of C6, and to the lower limb of L5; the patient is asked to indicate when they feel the contact.

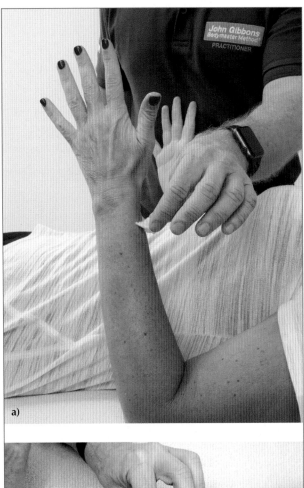

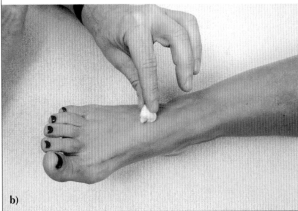

Figure 6.5: *Application of light touch to: (a) C6 dermatome; (b) L5 dermatome.*

Sharpness/Bluntness (Pinprick)

The sharpness/bluntness test entails the use of a dedicated neurological testing pin, where one tip is sharp and the other tip is blunt.

- Use the sternal area of the chest to establish a baseline for sharpness before you begin.
- Follow the same progression as for testing light touch, with the patient's eyes closed, and compare both upper limbs.

- Alternate between using sharp and blunt tips of the testing pin on each area of the dermatomes; the same applies to each limb. Ask the patient to report a sharp or blunt feeling, and note down any reduced or increased sensation.

Figure 6.6(a) and (b) demonstrates the application of a sharp or blunt tip to the upper limb dermatome of C8 and also to the lower limb dermatome of L4. The patient is asked to say what type of sensation they feel (either sharp or blunt).

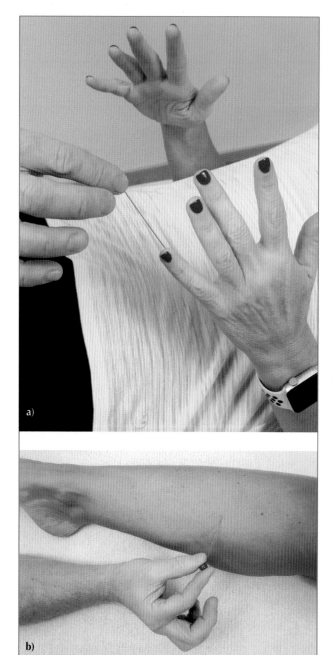

Figure 6.6: *Application of a sharp or blunt tip to: (a) C8 dermatome; (b) L4 dermatome.*

Temperature

This technique for testing temperature is often overlooked, but it can be important (Figure 6.7).

- Ideally, a small bowl of cold water and a small bowl of warm water would be available for use.
- Place a spoon in the cold water, apply to the patient, and repeat using the warm water.
- Ask the patient if they perceive the spoon to be cold and then warm.
- Another approach, and a simple and practical option, is to touch the patient with the end of a patella hammer, as it will feel cold.
- Compare the quality of temperature sensation of the specific dermatomes.

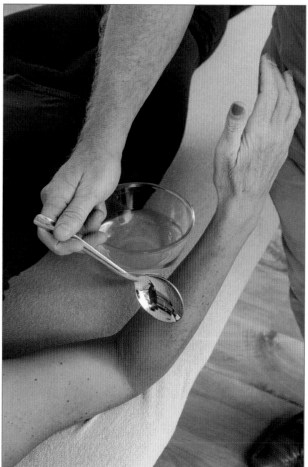

Figure 6.7: *The contact of a cold spoon (after immersion in cold water).*

Vibration

Vibratory sensation can be diminished in peripheral neuropathy (diabetes) and also in spinal cord disease, so it is important that one is familiar with this procedure. A tuning fork (Figure 6.8) is used for this technique, and the fork will need to be tapped to ensure that it is vibrating.

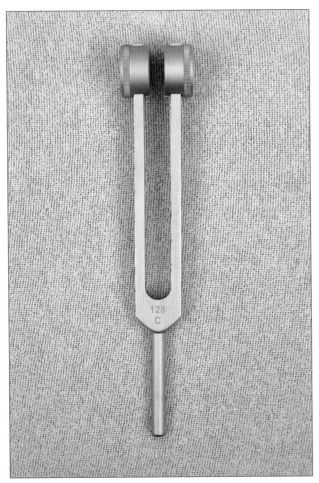

Figure 6.8: *Tuning fork.*

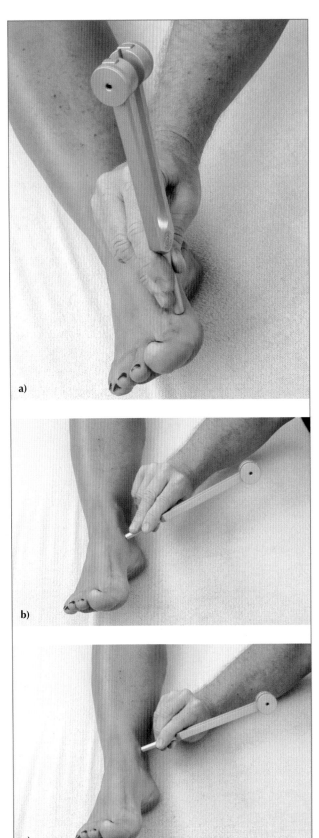

Figure 6.9: *Application of the tuning fork to: (a) MTP joint of hallux; (b) navicular tuberosity; (c) medial malleolus.*

- Place the non-vibration end of the tuning fork directly on the sternum to begin with, so that the patient can feel the start of the sensation and also when the fork stops vibrating.
- Next, place the fork on one of the interphalangeal (IP) joints of the hallux or pollex, and then ask the patient if they can feel the vibration.
- If no vibration is sensed, place the fork on the metatarsophalangeal (MTP) joint of the hallux and repeat (Figure 6.9). Again, if no vibration is perceived, keep moving proximally to the next joint or bone (navicular tuberosity), then to the medial malleolus, and work proximally to the tibial tuberosity, etc. Repeat the test until the patient is able to detect the vibratory sensation.

Joint Position Sense

Joint position sense (proprioception) can be tested in a simple manner by asking the patient, with their eyes closed, to say when they feel you performing a flexion or extension motion of their joints (Figure 6.10).

Dermatome testing – upper limb

Dermatome testing – lower limb

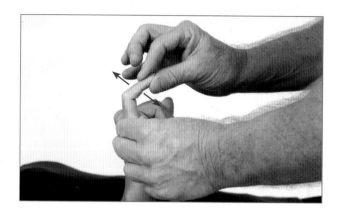

Figure 6.10: *Joint position sense: the practitioner flexes and extends the finger of the patient (eyes closed).*

7

Motor Testing—Myotomes

■ Examination of the Motor System (Myotome)

A *myotome* is a group of muscles innervated by a single nerve root.

The information set out in this chapter is possibly some of the most valuable text within this book; however, most therapists might simply browse through it and not really understand the importance of testing the myotomes. I cannot emphasize enough that muscle strength testing is an integral part of the neurological assessment process with patients, as it can assist the therapist in identifying where a specific lesion is located.

I remember watching a Canadian chiropractor assess and treat the Oxford rowing team, and his main evaluation of the athletes involved asking them to contract certain muscles while he resisted the motion. His findings dictated which area of the body he would then treat; for example, if the resisted motion testing procedures for shoulder abduction and elbow flexion resulted in, let's say, a grade 3 on the power scale (see Table 7.1 in

the "Power Testing" section below), this would indicate that the C5 myotome was weaker than normal. The chiropractor would then adjust (manipulate) the levels C4 and C5, because the exiting nerve root between these two vertebrae is C5, and when the chiropractor tested the myotome of C5, this proved to be weaker. After having done the adjustment, he would retest the power of the two movements, and hopefully this would now be graded as a "5" (see Table 7.1), which is classified as *normal power*.

When I watched this chiropractor at work, I was honestly very impressed, and even now I still use some of what I witnessed in my own treatment protocols. The problem is, there are only a few skilled therapists who can perform the manipulation technique, because it is a skill that takes many years to master. However, my goal here is not to teach you how to manipulate, but rather to help you understand the role of testing the myotomes, so that you know the level(s) of the spine in which the underlying problem(s) might lie. Every therapist has the ability to learn these unique techniques that I am about to show you.

■ Power Testing

Put simply, we ask the patient to perform a specific joint motion, then to hold that position (isometrically) while the practitioner tries to overcome the movement. This procedure is effective for testing, in a natural way, the muscles that are related to a particular motion. For example, when the patient is asked to resist shoulder abduction, the muscles responsible for this motion are naturally the deltoids and the smaller, but more important, supraspinatus muscle; however, it is the specific level of the C5 nerve root that is *allowing* the ability of these

Table 7.1: Grading system for the myotomes.

0	No muscle contraction is visible
1	Muscle contraction is visible but there is no movement of the joint
2	Active joint movement is possible with gravity eliminated
3	Movement can overcome gravity but not resistance from the examiner
4	The muscle group can overcome gravity and move against some resistance from the examiner
5	Full and normal power against resistance

muscles to contract. If the motion is just weaker, this could indicate a possible nerve root problem, but if the motion is both *weaker* and *painful*, then the patient might have torn their rotator cuff muscle group (supraspinatus mainly). In the case of weak and painful motion, we can also ask the patient to resist against elbow flexion, because the biceps and brachialis muscles are also innervated by the level C5 through the musculocutaneous nerve. If *both* elbow flexion and shoulder abduction are weaker, we know the problem lies with the nerve root of C5.

Just to clarify, the muscle group being tested is used to identify the subsequent nerve root that is related to the corresponding myotome. The examiner will try to overpower that muscle group, and any weakness found during the muscle testing procedures could indicate a problem with the corresponding nerve root. Muscle power is ranked from 0 to 5 according to the grading system in Table 7.1.

Myotome Maps

Tables 7.2 and 7.3 present the specific spinal nerve root levels for the myotomes of the upper and lower limbs.

Table 7.2: Map of the myotomes of the upper limb.

Myotome location—upper limb	Spinal level
Cervical flexion/extension	C1/C2
Cervical lateral flexion	C3
Shoulder elevation	C4
Shoulder abduction and elbow flexion	C5
Elbow flexion and wrist extension	C6
Elbow extension, wrist flexion, and finger extension	C7
Finger flexion	C8
Finger abduction and adduction	T1

Table 7.3: Map of the myotomes of the lower limb.

Myotome location—lower limb	Spinal level
Hip flexion	L2
Knee extension	L3
Ankle dorsiflexion	L4
Great toe (hallux) extension	L5
Ankle plantar flexion/eversion and hip extension	S1
Knee flexion	S2

■ Part 1: Upper Limb Myotome Testing

1. Cervical Flexion/Extension—C1/C2 Myotomes

- Place your hand on the forehead of the seated patient.
- Ask the patient to flex their cervical spine against your resistance (Figure 7.1(a)).
- Applying your hand on the patient's occipital bone.
- Ask the patient to extend their cervical spine against your resistance (Figure 7.1(b)).

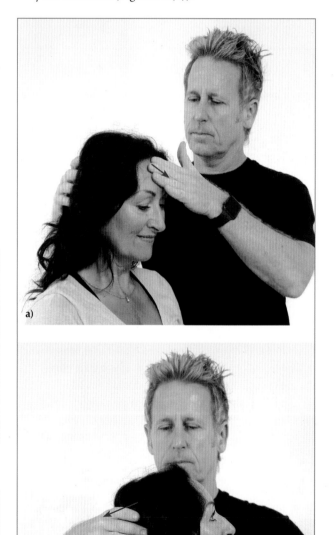

Figure 7.1: (a) Resisted cervical flexion. (b) Resisted cervical extension.

2. Cervical Lateral Flexion—C3 Myotome

- Place your hand on the lateral side of the forehead of the seated patient.
- Ask the patient to laterally flex their cervical spine against your resistance (Figure 7.2).

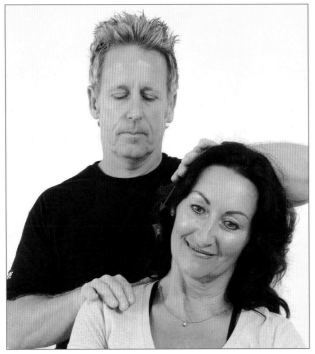

Figure 7.2: *Resisted cervical lateral flexion.*

3. Shoulder Elevation—C4 Myotome

- Place your hand on the top of the shoulder of the seated patient.
- Ask the patient to elevate their shoulder girdle against your resistance (Figure 7.3).

4. Shoulder Abduction and Elbow Flexion—C5 Myotome

- Place your hands just above the elbows of the seated patient.
- Ask the patient to abduct their shoulders (or one side at a time) to 90 degrees against your resistance (Figure 7.4(a)).
- Place your hands on the lower part of the patient's forearms.
- Ask the patient to flex their elbows to 90 degrees against your resistance (Figure 7.4(b)).

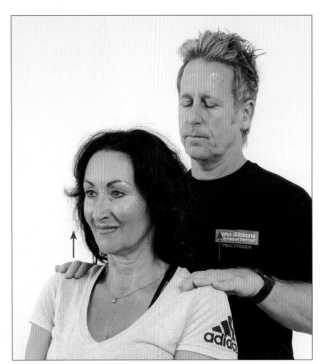

Figure 7.3: *Resisted shoulder elevation.*

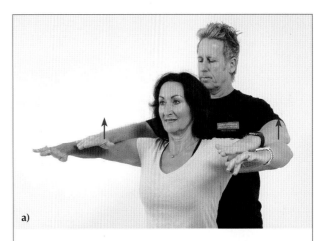

a)

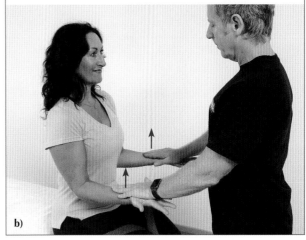

b)

Figure 7.4: *(a) Resisted shoulder abduction. (b) Resisted elbow flexion.*

5. Elbow Flexion and Wrist Extension—C6 Myotome

Elbow flexion has already been covered (see Figure 7.4(b)), but just to recap, the patient is asked to flex their elbows to 90 degrees, as will test the C5 and C6 myotomes. To test wrist extension (mainly the C6 myotome):

- Place your hand on the top of the patient's hand.
- Ask the patient to extend their wrist against your resistance (Figure 7.5).

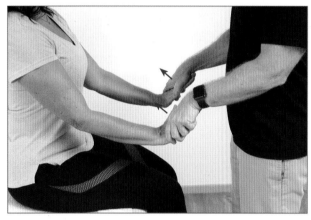

Figure 7.5: *Resisted wrist extension.*

6. Elbow Extension, Wrist Flexion, and Finger Extension—C7 Myotome

Elbow extension:

- Place your hand on the distal medial forearm of the seated patient.
- Ask the patient to flex their elbows to 90 degrees and to then extend their elbows against your resistance (Figure 7.6(a)).

Wrist flexion:

- Place your hand under the patient's hand.
- Ask the patient to flex their wrist against your resistance (Figure 7.6(b)).

Finger extension:

- Place your hand over the patient's fingers.
- Ask the patient to extend their fingers against your resistance (Figure 7.6(c)).

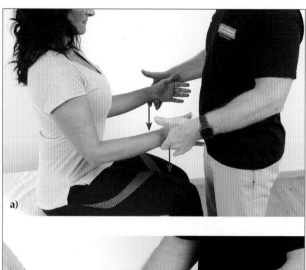

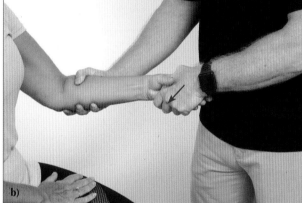

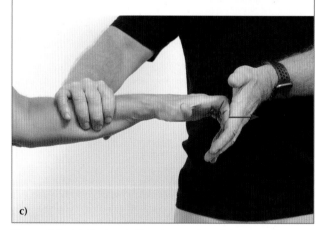

Figure 7.6: *(a) Resisted elbow extension. (b) Resisted wrist flexion. (c) Resisted finger extension.*

7. Finger Flexion—C8 Myotome

- Place your hand under the seated patient's fingers.
- Ask the patient to flex their fingers against your resistance (Figure 7.7).

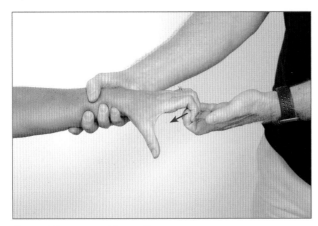

Figure 7.7: *Resisted finger flexion.*

8. Finger Abduction and Adduction— T1 Myotome

- Interlock your fingers with the fingers of the seated patient.
- Ask the patient to abduct and adduct their fingers against your resistance (Figure 7.8).

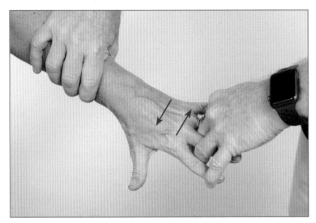

Figure 7.8: *Resisted finger abduction and adduction.*

Myotome testing – upper limb

■ Part 2: Lower Limb Myotome Testing

In the majority of procedures in this section, the patient is mainly in a supine position, although the tests can be performed in a seated position. I personally find it easier to assess this way, and for some myotome tests, I ask the patient to turn over and adopt a prone position.

1. Hip Flexion—L2 Myotome

- Instruct the patient to adopt a supine position.
- Flex the patient's hip and knee to 90 degrees, and support the area above the knee.
- Ask the patient to flex their hip against your resistance (Figure 7.9).

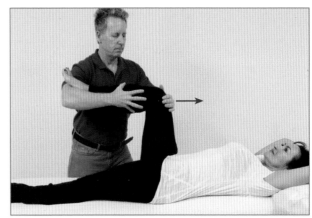

Figure 7.9: *Resisted hip flexion.*

2. Knee Extension—L3 Myotome

- Place your bent leg underneath the patient's knee.
- Ask the patient to extend their knee against your resistance (Figure 7.10).

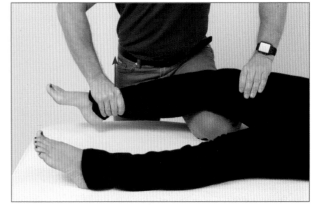

Figure 7.10: *Resisted knee extension.*

3. Ankle Dorsiflexion—L4 Myotome

- Instruct the patient to adopt a supine position, and place your hand over their foot.

- Ask the patient to dorsiflex and also invert their ankle against your resistance (Figure 7.11). This activates the tibialis anterior.

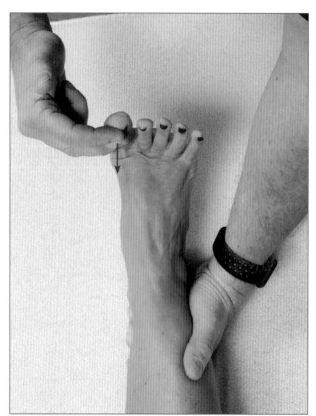

Figure 7.12: *Resisted great toe extension.*

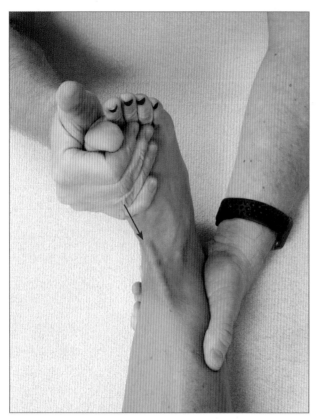

Figure 7.11: *Resisted ankle dorsiflexion and inversion.*

4. Great Toe (Hallux) Extension—L5 Myotome

- Instruct the patient to adopt a supine position, and place your fingers under their great toe.
- Ask the patient to extend their great toe against your resistance (Figure 7.12). This activates the extensor hallucis longus (EHL).

5. Ankle Plantar Flexion—S1 Myotome

- Instruct the patient to adopt a supine position, and place your hand under the patient's foot.
- Ask the patient to plantarflex their ankle against your resistance (Figure 7.13). This activates the triceps surae muscles—gastrocnemius and soleus.

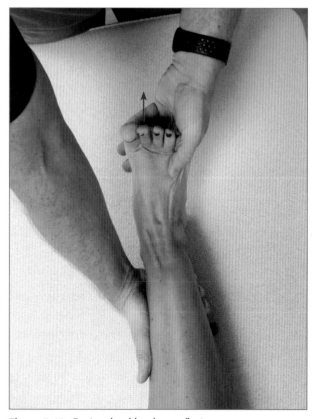

Figure 7.13: *Resisted ankle plantar flexion.*

6. Ankle Eversion—S1 Myotome

- Instruct the patient to adopt a supine position, and place your hand over the top of the outside edge of their foot.
- Ask the patient to evert their ankle against your resistance (Figure 7.14). This activates the fibulares.

Myotome testing – lower limb

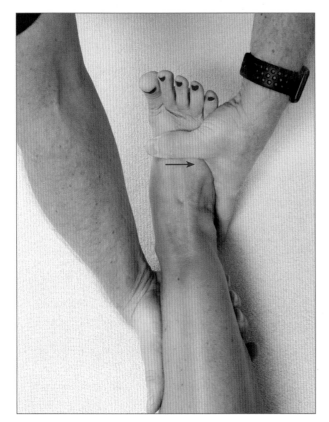

Figure 7.14: *Resisted ankle eversion.*

7. Hip Extension—S1 Myotome

- Instruct the patient to adopt a prone position.
- Flex the patient's knee to 90 degrees, and place your hand on the back of the patient's leg, just above their knee.
- Ask the patient to extend their hip toward the ceiling against your resistance (Figure 7.15).

8. Knee Flexion—S2 Myotome

- Instruct the patient to adopt a prone position.
- Bend the patient's knee slightly, and place your hand on the back of the patient's leg, just above their ankle.
- Ask the patient to flex their knee against your resistance (Figure 7.16).

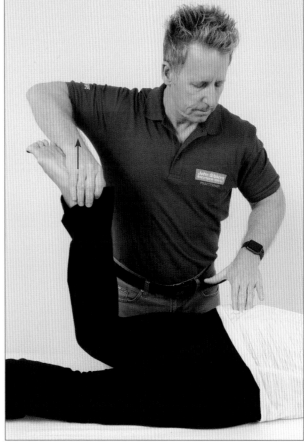

Figure 7.15: *Resisted hip extension.*

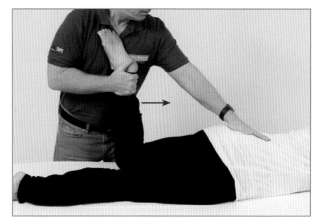

Figure 7.16: *Resisted knee flexion.*

■ Simple Testing Procedures for the L4–S1 Myotomes

In reality, disc pathology will only affect two main levels, namely L4/L5 and L5/S1; the three nerve roots affected will be those of L4, L5, and S1. A potentially easier way to ascertain the ability of the myotomes, therefore, is to run through the following simple tests, as they can rule out any obvious condition.

L4/L5—Quick Test

To rule out an L4/L5 issue, ask the patient to stand up and try to walk on their *heels* or to simply lift their toes off the ground (Figure 7.17); this extension action entails dorsiflexion of the ankle. I can guarantee that if there is an L4 or L5 nerve root problem, the patient will not be able to perform any of these extension movements.

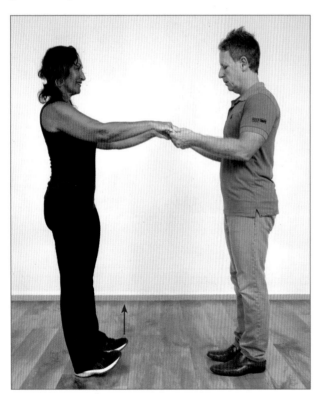

Figure 7.17: *Walking on the heels to rule out any L4 or L5 condition.*

S1—Quick Test

To rule out an S1 issue, ask the patient to walk on their *toes* (Figure 7.18(a)); this is a plantar flexion motion of the ankle, but with more resistance. Ask the patient to now perform a single-leg calf raise on the good side, and to try to repeat this on the problem side (Figure 7.18(b)).

I can guarantee that if there is an S1 nerve root problem, the patient will not be able to do any of these calf-raising movements on the problem side. Please ensure that there is no rupture present of the Achilles tendon, as this too will cause weakness in the calf raise.

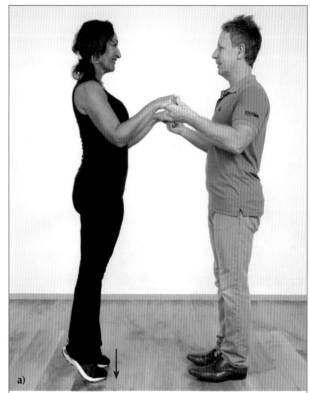

a)

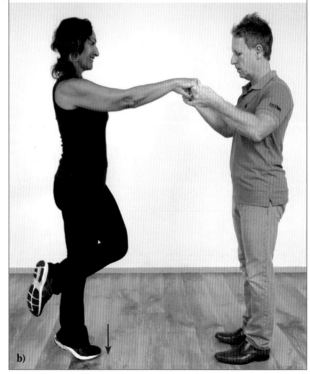

b)

Figure 7.18: *(a) Walking on the toes. (b) Single-leg calf raise to rule out any S1 condition.*

Standing tests for L4, L5 & S1

■ Conclusion

Remember that myotome testing is just one integral part of a neurological examination performed by the practitioner. It is like a adding a small piece to a jigsaw puzzle: hopefully, the picture becomes a little clearer as you continue to add the pieces. It is worth remembering that most of the therapists reading this book (including myself) will not have undergone the same training as neurologists. However, it is just as important for us to be able to decipher what we have ascertained during a neurological examination, and, more crucially, to know what are we going to do about it if we find a problem.

8

Intervertebral Disc Anatomy and Conditions

■ Introduction

Whenever I say to one of my patients that I consider a disc might be the source of their problem (especially if they are presenting with what I believe to be referred pain such as sciatica), I personally believe that they naturally assume that their disc has *slipped* or *moved* somewhere. (By the way the "slipping" myth is incorrect, as the disc does not slip anywhere, even though it is commonly called a *slipped disc*.) The problem I encounter now is that they naturally expect me, as an osteopath, to *crack* or *manipulate* the disc back into its normal position; this is the general consensus of some patients' views of what osteopaths and chiropractors do—they manipulate the disc back into place. Hopefully, after reading the following text, you will see that this is not the case, as disc conditions can be rather complex. But just to be clear—*discs do not slip.*

Whichever way you look at it, disc pathology will be present for all of us at some point in our lives, and for some it will occur sooner rather than later. For patients who have referred pain (e.g., sciatica), then an underlying disc condition is probably near the top of the ladder as a potential causative factor, although there are a multitude of reasons (not just disc related) why patients suffer sciatic pain. It therefore makes perfect sense to spend some time discussing disc anatomy, function, and of course conditions that can manifest within these unique and amazing structures.

I would imagine that many therapists consider disc problems to be linked to those individuals who are not very active, who are overweight, and who have weak

core muscles. That might be true for some patients; however, most of my patients at the University of Oxford are very fit athletes between the ages of 18 and 30. I am of the belief that it is not always "sport" in general that causes problems, but rather the continual training sessions. For example, I have been the resident osteopath for the Oxford University rowing team (Boat Race) for many years, and typically each member of the team will spend most mornings on a rowing machine for approximately 60–90 minutes, as well as each afternoon and weekends rowing on the River Thames. When I see an oarsperson with back pain that I consider to be disc related, it might be that they bent down to pick something up from the floor, such as an oar (or even a pen), and felt their back "go," in which case their pain was not caused by the actual specifics of the rowing motion. The problem they have now, though, is that any rowing motion (bending and extending with rotation) will exacerbate the pain, whether they are using a rowing machine or rowing on the river. No doubt the continual flexion and rotation of the rowing motion has predisposed them and contributed to the overall disc condition and the simple action of bending to pick something up (or perhaps even a bout of coughing or sneezing) ultimately caused the disc to fail and to subsequently bulge.

When I see patients at the clinic with lower back pain, the last thing I consider my patient to have is a disc problem. However, if my patient has lower back pain and some buttock and leg pain, and they also mention that simple motions like coughing or sneezing or even sitting or bending forward increase their symptoms, then my hypothesis dramatically changes.

In this chapter I would like to discuss the anatomy of a disc, the symptoms it can present, and the specific differences between a bulging/protruding disc and a prolapsed disc.

Even though human bodies are all very similar in terms of structure and function, everybody is a unique individual, and some symptoms will vary between patients. Nevertheless, you can use the following signs and symptoms as a sort of tick box list in establishing whether your patient might have an underlying lumbar spine disc condition:

- There is some history of bending with a rotational component, or simply a cough or a sneeze.
- A couple of days after an initial injury, pain begins to develop in the area of the buttocks and/or leg, as well as in the shoulder, arm, and hand (if a cervical disc).
- There is an aversion to sitting for long periods, which makes driving very uncomfortable.
- Standing for long periods brings on discomfort, or sleeping is difficult because of night pain.
- Stiffness is felt, and buttock/leg pain increases, when bending forward to touch the toes or simply putting on socks in the morning.
- Bending backward increases the pain (as the action can potentially catch the posterior aspect of the disc bulge).
- Coughing, sneezing, or defecating (bearing down motion) increases the symptoms.
- Lower back is generally stiff and potentially painful upon waking in the morning.
- A particular discomfort is felt when sitting, with the impression of squirming in the chair seat. Adopting a position of ease is difficult.
- After lower back symptoms have eased off (which typically happens), buttock/leg pain usually lingers. (It is worth mentioning that some individuals have no history of back pain.)
- There is an inability to plantar- or dorsiflex the ankle on the painful leg (specific nerve dependent). (The disc is contacting the nerve root, causing weakness of the related muscles.)
- Slump test or straight leg raise test (SLR) is positive.
- Deep tendon reflex (DTR) of L4, L5, or S1 is reduced.

■ Intervertebral Disc Anatomy

Between adjacent vertebrae there is a structure known as an *intervertebral disc*, and these unique structures separate the vertebral bodies of the spine (Figure 8.1). The disc is

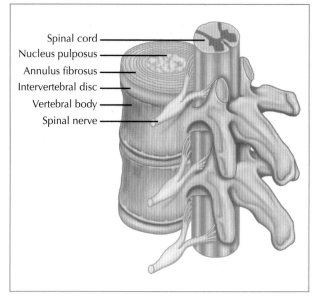

Figure 8.1: *Anatomy of an intervertebral disc.*

made up mainly of fibrocartilage, and in total we have 23 of these soft-tissue structures located within the human vertebral column. The disc has principally two layers—a soft inner layer and a hard outer layer.

The inner layer of a disc comprises a water-based gelatinous mass, known as the *nucleus pulposus*, with an attachment to the vertebral bodies, called the *vertebral end plate*. The nucleus pulposus contains mainly water, giving it the ability to act as a modified shock absorber every time the spinal column moves. The water composition unfortunately decreases with age, which contributes to the progressive decrease in our height as we get older.

The outer layer of a disc consists of a tough fibrous shell, known as the *annulus fibrosus*, and between shell structure and the inner nucleus pulposus there are individual fibrocartilaginous concentric layers, called *lamellae*, which increase the disc's shock-absorption capability. The ring-like appearance of the lamellae assist in giving the annulus its strength, as well as maintaining the water-based gelatinous fluid within the nucleus pulposus.

A healthy disc is very flexible. As we get older, however, the natural degenerative processes and other factors such as gravity and trauma will subsequently cause the disc to become compressed and hence stiffer, which makes the disc potentially more susceptible to injury. The center of the disc starts to lose its water content within the nucleus, a process that will naturally make the disc less elastic and less effective as a cushion or shock absorber. Furthermore, this cumulative and compressive force reduces the amount of much-needed nutrition and oxygen from entering the disc. Nutrients are necessary for the disc to stay healthy; without an adequate supply, the overall problem of disc degeneration is perpetuated.

Intervertebral discs are truly amazing structures, like all living tissue, and are made up of cells composed of the protein aggrecan (a proteoglycan). Located within these cells are tiny sponges, which are considered to be able to carry approximately 500 times their own weight of water. Over time, these unique cells eventually die, and so the water content within the nucleus will naturally reduce; this process will eventually lead to a condition called *degenerative disc disease* (DDD).

A disc is kept alive by the connection to the vertebral body through *vertebral end plates*. These plate structures have been likened to the parts of a tire: the inner nucleus is the air within the tire, the outer annulus is the tire's strong walls, and the tread of the tire forms the vertebral end plates. The discs are mainly *avascular* (lack of blood) structures, but are hydrated through diffusion by the vertebral bodies and subsequently by the end plates (Figure 8.2). The nerve supply derives mainly from the sinuvertebral nerves and is responsible for innervation of the outer periphery of the intervertebral disc.

Nerve roots exit the spinal canal through small passageways between the vertebrae and the discs: such a passageway is known as an *intervertebral foramen*. Pain and other symptoms can develop when the inner fluid from a damaged disc pushes into the spinal canal or nerve roots as they exit within the intervertebral foramen—a condition commonly referred to as a *herniated intervertebral disc* or *prolapsed intervertebral disc* (PID).

■ Intervertebral Disc Conditions

Disc Herniation

I would like to keep it simple in one respect, so one way of looking at any type of disc bulge is to say it is essentially a weakness in the outer covering of the shell (annulus fibrosus) that allows the soft contents inside (nucleus pulposus) to migrate outward and potentially toward the exiting spinal nerve roots. This is basically the first stage of DDD. I regard a *herniated* or *prolapsed disc* as a natural progression from a bulge or a protrusion, where the annulus has become weaker and can actually tear, allowing the nucleus to migrate even further toward the spinal nerves.

Some textbooks refer to herniated discs as *bulging discs*, *protruding discs*, *prolapsed discs*, or even *slipped discs*. These terms are derived from the nature of the action of

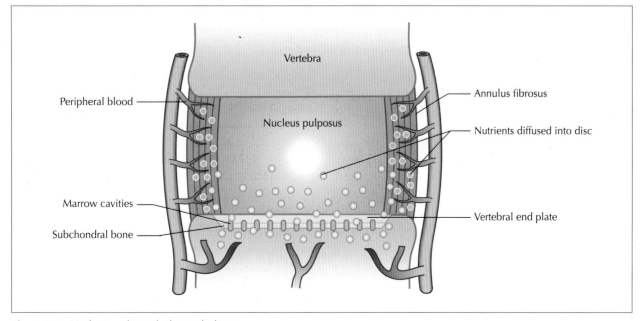

Figure 8.2: *Hydration through the end plates.*

the gel-like content of the nucleus pulposus being forced out of the center of the disc. Just to clarify, the disc itself does not actually slip; however, the nucleus pulposus tissue located in the center of the disc can be placed under so much pressure that it can cause the annulus fibrosus to herniate or even rupture (see Figure 8.3). The severity of disc herniation may cause the bulging tissue to press against one or more of the spinal nerves and/or the posterior longitudinal ligament, which can cause local and/or radicular pain, numbness, or weakness to the areas of the lower back, buttocks, and lower limb if a lumbar disc is involved. If it is a question of a cervical disc, the patient might perceive pain within the neck, shoulder, arm, and hand.

Discs and the Toothpaste Analogy

Please do not quote me on this analogy, but I personally like to think of a disc as a "tube of toothpaste" with the cap still tightly on. If you simply squeeze one end of the tube, the toothpaste (fluid) will migrate to the other end, and vice versa; the contents are still maintained within the tube and there is no seepage, but you will notice a bulge at the end of the tube because you have squeezed the opposite end. Now, if you take the cap completely off the tube of toothpaste and squeeze the tube, the contents will obviously come out of the end.

Let us think about this concept a little bit more and relate it to the subject of this book and the nerves (Figure 8.3).

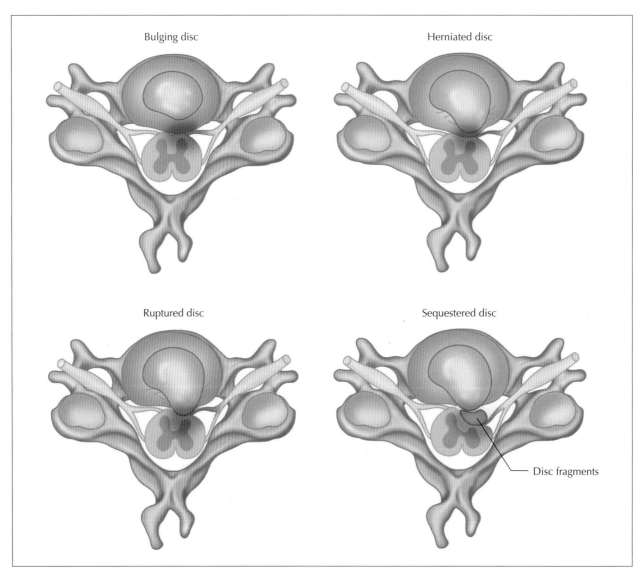

Figure 8.3: *Various disc conditions and the contact with the nerve root.*

Imagine the paste as the *nucleus pulposus*, and the outer shell of the tube as the *annulus fibrosus*; hopefully, you are on the same wavelength as me. Now, suppose the cap is on but almost coming off (if it takes five turns to lock the cap and five turns to lift it off, say for argument's sake it is on two turns); if you squeeze the tube, you might notice the end bulging (as in a bulging disc). If you squeeze the tube hard enough, however, the toothpaste (fluid) might actually be seen to ooze out around the base of the cap; this might be likened to a *protrusion*. If the cap actually comes off altogether, this is what you would call a *herniated* or *prolapsed disc*, and if some of the toothpaste detaches itself, and is now separate from the rest, this would be referred to as a *sequestered disc*. Hopefully, this all makes sense!

Typically, when a patient lifts something from the floor, most of the pressure is applied to the anterior part of the disc. This will push the nucleus pulposus posteriorly against the posterior aspect of the annulus fibrosus, which incidentally is thinner than the anterior part, and so is more susceptible to injury. The majority of cervical spine disc herniations will occur at the cervical segments C4–5, C5–6, or C6–7 (see Figure 9.1). The nerve compression caused by the contact with the disc contents will possibly result in perceived pain (radicular) along

either the C5, C6, or C7 nerve root pathways, as shown in Figure 8.4.

With regard to the lumbar spine, the most common areas for disc herniations are the lumbar segments L4–L5 or L5–S1, and approximately 85–95% of them will occur here. The nerve compression caused by the contact with the disc contents will possibly result in perceived pain along the L4, L5, or S1 nerve root pathways, as shown in Figure 8.5.

Note: It is not the nerve emerging through the space associated with the prolapsing disc, but the **next nerve down**. This is because the nerve in that space emerges high in the intervertebral foramen and thus hits the nerve that is moving anteriorly to emerge through the next space; therefore, the L4/5 disc will contact the **L5** nerve root and not usually the L4 exiting nerve. The same applies in the case of the L5/S1 disc prolapse, as this will typically contact the **S1** nerve root, although if the prolapse is severe enough it can contact both nerve roots.

In the cervical region, however, it is the actual nerve emerging through the intervertebral foramen that is being contacted by the prolapse and **not** the one below; thus, a C4/5 prolapse will only contact the exiting **C5** nerve root.

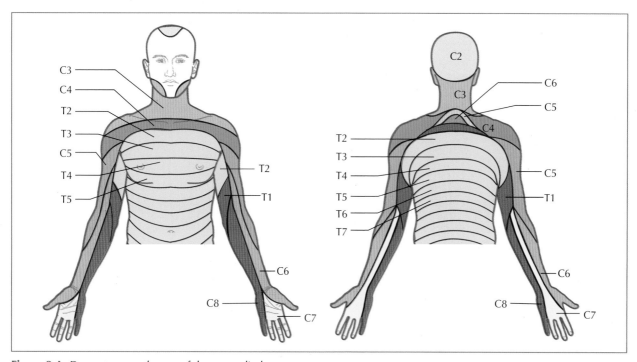

Figure 8.4: *Dermatome pathways of the upper limb.*

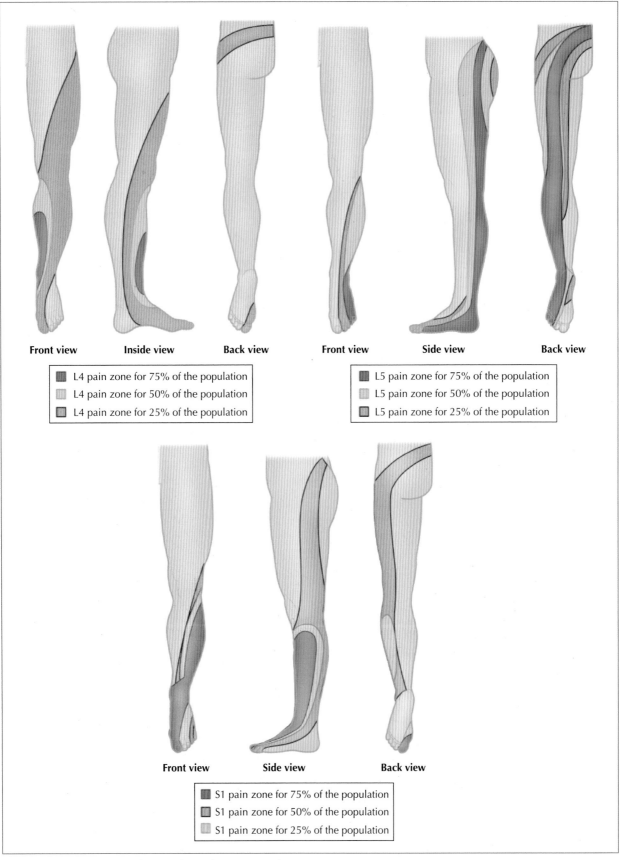

Figure 8.5: *Dermatome pathways of pain for L4, L5, and S1 nerve roots.*

Central Disc Prolapse and Cauda Equina Syndrome

A large prolapsed disc within the cervical spine can contact the actual spinal cord and subsequently cause upper motor neuron symptoms. An example of this condition will be explained in Case Study 9.1 in Chapter 9.

What I would like to mention, however, is a central disc prolapse located within the lumbar spine, as this can contact the end of the spinal cord, which has formed bundles of nerves called the *cauda equina*, resembling the tail of a horse (see Figure 8.6). This rare condition can cause a devastating neurological disorder called *cauda equina syndrome* (CES). If this condition is not diagnosed and treated in time, then there can be serious consequences. Typically, the patient complains of urinary or rectal incontinence, with saddle anesthesia as well as bilateral leg pain and associated weakness. Urgent surgery within 48 hours from the initial onset of symptoms is required in order to correct this serious medical condition.

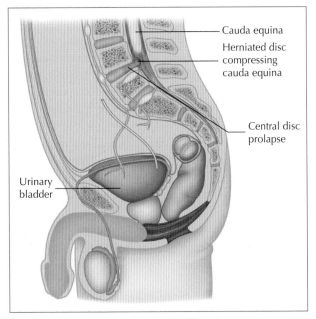

Figure 8.6: *Central disc prolapse and cauda equina syndrome.*

Degenerative Disc Disease

DDD tends to be linked to the aging process and refers to a syndrome in which a painful disc causes associated chronic lower back pain, which can radiate to the hip

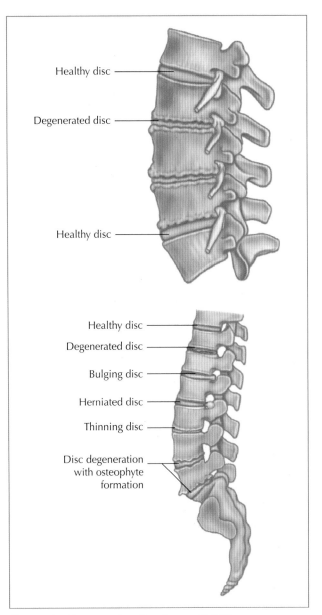

Figure 8.7: *Degenerative disc disease (DDD).*

region (Figure 8.7). The condition generally occurs as a consequence of some form of injury to the lower back and the associated structures, such as the intervertebral discs. A sustained injury can cause an inflammatory process and subsequent weakness of the outer shell of the disc (annulus fibrosus), which will then have a pronounced effect on the inner substance (nucleus pulposus). This reactive mechanism will create excessive movement, because the disc can no longer control the motion of the vertebral bodies located above and below the disc. The excessive movement, combined with the natural inflammatory response, will produce chemicals that irritate the local area, which commonly produce symptoms of chronic lower back pain.

DDD has been shown to cause an increase in the number of clusters of chondrocytes (cells that form the cartilaginous matrix and consist mainly of collagen) in the annulus fibrosus (consisting of fibrocartilage). Over a prolonged period of time, the inner gelatinous nucleus pulposus can change to fibrocartilage, and it has been shown that the outer annulus can become damaged in areas that allow some of the nucleus material to herniate through, causing the disc to shrink and eventually leading to the formation of bony spurs called *osteophytes*.

Unlike the muscles in the back, the discs of the lumbar spine do not have a natural blood supply and therefore cannot heal themselves; the painful symptoms of DDD can therefore become chronic, eventually leading to further problems, such as disc herniation, facet joint pain, nerve root compression, spondylolysis (defect of the pars interarticularis), and spinal stenosis (narrowing of the spinal canal).

■ Types of Pain

Shooting Pain/Radicular Pain

Another name for a shooting-type pain either in the arm or the leg is *radicular pain*. Sciatica is the most common type of radicular pain and tends to be sharper, band like, and electric in nature, and follows the nerve root dermatome pattern. The mechanism of radicular pain is considered to originate from inflammation of the nerve root or compression of the dorsal root ganglion (DRG).

Radiculopathy Pain

Radiculopathy tends to coexist with radicular pain. Radiculopathy, however, is classified as either a neurological loss of sensation or a change in sensation; typically, these present as numbness and tingling and/ or motor loss, where the patient will demonstrate loss of strength/weakness of the associated muscles and reduced reflexes. Radiculopathy is generally caused by the compression of nerve roots. The most common causes of both types of radicular symptom are conditions mainly caused by spinal disc herniation (by far the most common cause). Pain can also result from hypertrophy of the spinal facet joints, osteophytes (bony spurs), and spinal stenosis (narrowing of the spinal or vertebral canal).

Referred Pain

Referred pain is the term used for pain that is perceived in an area of the body distant from the original site. Think about a heart attack (myocardial infarction), for example: the pain is felt by patients not only in the central chest area (origin), but possibly also at distant sites such as the jaw, back, arm, and hand—hence the term *referred*. In Chapter 11, on differential diagnosis, I will discuss many referred pain syndromes, such as how the gallbladder "refers" pain to the shoulder and how the process of referral works.

Axial Pain

Typically, *axial pain* is generally thought of as "mechanical" in nature, and tends to be local to the actual source. This type of pain can be dull and aching, but may have a referred component to it as well. For example, the lumbar facet joints can give local back pain, especially during particular movements such as exercises; however, the facets can also refer pain to the buttock and leg, so it is not always that easy to localize the source.

Another example of axial pain is the following. If a patient has axial neck or axial lower back pain, in these cases the pain is generally caused by a structural component within the neck or lower back, and the pain is also perceived by the patient in those areas.

■ Where Is the Patient's Pain?

Let us take the cervical spine as an example of a potential location of your patient's presenting symptoms. It is important to try to ascertain the cause, because if the patient says to you that their pain is localized within the neck region, then it is probably going to be *axial neck pain*. If, on the other hand, the patient mentions that it is difficult to locate the pain, because it seems more widespread than just local to the neck, and is duller and achier in nature, then it is probably *referred pain*. However, were the patient to say that the pain is sharper, stabbing, and band like, then naturally it is likely to be *radicular pain*.

Just to clarify: if radicular symptoms are suspected from the cervical spine at the level of the C5 nerve root, typically the patient will perceive altered sensations in the area of the lateral shoulder and lateral ante-cubital fossa. C6 nerve root radicular symptoms are most often associated with the first digit (thumb) and forearm, and those of the C7 nerve root with the third digit (middle finger). The C8 nerve root affects the fifth digit (little finger), and the T1 nerve root presents radicular symptoms in the region of the medial ante-cubital fossa.

■ Case Study

I have always naturally been particularly stiff and very inflexible, particularly in my lower back and hips, and I can recall being this way as far back as my memory allows. I could never touch my toes, and when I joined the British Army at 16 years old, I remember failing the flexibility tests. I think this is rather funny in some respect, especially as I used to teach flexibility sessions for the crew of the Oxford Boat Race team!

Case Study 8.1 is actually about me and a problem that started in 2008 and went on for more than three months. Being an osteopath who suffered from lumbar spine and leg pain was not a very good marketing strategy, especially for business.

CASE STUDY 8.1

Many years ago, I decided to modify the fishpond in my garden, and after five hours of huge quantities of earth and rock shifting, my lower back felt very stiff. The next morning when I woke up, I felt like an old man, unable to move very well in bed because of the pain and stiffness in my lower back region. I eventually (very slowly) made my way to the pain cabinet and took some anti-inflammatories as well as some pain-killers (ibuprofen and paracetamol). The pain slowly subsided a little and I was sort of able to go through my daily routine. A few days later, I started to feel some numbness in the lateral side of my left tibia, but also perceived a particularly sharp pain in my left quadriceps and tensor fasciae latae (TFL) muscles. This seemed to progressively get worse over a few days, to the point that I could not sleep on my back in a comfortable position and walking to the shop was unbearable owing to the pain in my left anterior thigh.

As an osteopath, I naturally "self-diagnosed" myself: I considered I had an L4/5 disc bulge that was pressing on my exiting L4 nerve. I also thought the bulge to be large enough to compress the L5 descending (traversing) nerve as well, mainly because of the dermatome distribution

in my lateral tibia. What was strange with me, though, was that my anterior thigh pain on a dermatome map was somewhere located between the L2 and L3 nerves, and there was no medial tibia pain (L4) at all. So, I was a bit confused, given that I also had excruciating pain in my left TFL, as well as groin pain on my left side. My overall conclusion was that my psoas must be involved, as the lumbar plexus penetrates the psoas muscle and was causing this muscle to produce a kind of protective spasm with a resultant referral pattern.

My deep tendon reflex of L4 was reduced to less than a 1+ (and still is, many years later). The muscle strength (myotome) of the left quadriceps muscles (knee extension) when tested was weaker, as was the strength of the left anterior tibialis muscle (ankle dorsiflexion). This confirmed to me that the problem was indeed a neurological one, and I thought it had manifested as a result of a disc bulge.

Strangely enough, I found that sitting was the most comfortable position for me, as I was to later find out; I much rather preferred sitting at my desk at 3am, emailing anyone and everyone to pass the time, to suffering the extreme pain in my quads when I attempted to lie down to sleep. This pain resulted in 58 consecutive disturbed nights, trying to sleep on the floor with my legs on the sofa (psoas position), as it was the only position that I could find that provided me with some pain relief, albeit for a few hours at a time, before I would sit and start emailing random people.

One week after an MRI self-referral (and a significant reduction in my bank account balance), it was confirmed that I had an L4/5 bulging disc that was just in contact with the L4 nerve root. I consulted a friend of mine who is a neurosurgeon, and almost immediately I asked him to operate on me, as I thought it was my only option. However, he said that he would prefer to wait and that, typically, the pain often subsides; moreover, as my disc bulge was laterally placed, he would have to remove a facet joint in order to get to the bulge. The effect of this over time on me would be to become less flexible, and to potentially cause me ongoing back pain. His advice was to avoid bending for nine months and let things settle down on their own.

After the prescription of codeine, diclofenac, tramadol, and anything else I could try, I decided that medication was not the answer for me. Basically, none of the prescribed pills really seemed to help my current symptoms.

So, what did I do? Well, I bought an inversion table, as I had researched the most effective way of treating disc pain. I used this table regularly (twice daily), and I do feel it helped to reduce my symptoms, on the basis that pain arises from a bulge that may be as little as 0.04″ (1mm) in the wrong direction. If the disc happens to be bulging away from the ligaments and nerves, there is either a reduction in pain or no pain at all. However, a bulge 1mm in the other direction results in considerable pain, and that is how it was with me: one day would be slightly better and another would be particularly painful.

Three months later and one and a half stone (10kg) lighter and very depressed, I started to improve, albeit very slowly, but things were nevertheless moving in the right direction.

At least I can now run again and have resumed training, although somewhat modified. Even today, I avoid lifting heavy objects and training with very heavy weights, and especially steer clear of movements like deadlifts etc. I am acutely aware that if the disc moves just 1mm in the wrong direction, I will feel it, but in particular it will remind me of the 58 nights lying on my back on the floor, with my legs over the sofa … not a good place to be!

Prognosis, Treatment, and Conclusion

As an osteopath, I have treated numerous patients with back pain, and I have referred a small number of them for an MRI scan, because I considered these particular patients to have suffered some form of disc condition. Approximately 10–20% of the patients I see with a disc condition that is confirmed by the MRI, I have referred to the neurosurgeon for a second opinion. The neurosurgeon will then decide what the best options are for the patient; in reality, the majority of the patients I refer to the surgeon will eventually have spinal surgery.

It is very difficult to say "what" is the best conservative treatment or even "what" is the best management of a disc bulge, as everybody will react slightly differently. My neurosurgeon friend's advice was to simply "not bend down for nine months and wait to see what nature will do." For me, like for others, that is very simple advice, and with the help of the inversion table, it actually helped reduce the presenting symptoms.

9

Anatomy, Function, and Assessment of the Cervical Spine

■ Cervical Spine Anatomy

The human cervical spine (Figure 9.1) has seven vertebrae (C1–7) and eight cervical nerves (C1–8), and an upper cervical complex comprising the atlas (C1) and the axis (C2). The lower cervical spine, comprising the remaining five cervical vertebrae C3 to C7 has structural features that are more typical of other spinal levels.

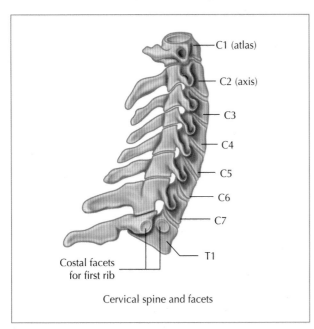

Figure 9.1: *Anatomy of the cervical spine.*

In functional terms, the cervical spine section of the vertebral column should also include the occipital condyles, which transfer the weight of the head to the uppermost cervical vertebra, C1. This highly specialized

vertebra, known as the *atlas* (Figure 9.2), is aptly named after the Titan Atlas in classical mythology, whose role was to support the whole world on his shoulders. The second cervical vertebra, C2, known as the *axis* (Figure 9.2), is also a specialized structure, since its function is mainly to assist in rotation of the head.

General Anatomy of a Vertebra

If you look at Figure 9.3, you will see the anatomical landmarks that are associated with a typical vertebra.

- Vertebral body
- Spinous process
- Transverse process
- Facet joint
- Intervertebral foramen
- Spinal canal
- Lamina
- Pedicle
- Intervertebral disc:
  - nucleus pulposus
  - annulus fibrosus

Facet Joints

Located within the cervical spine are the facet joints, anatomically known as the *zygapophyseal joints* (Figure 9.4); these structures can be responsible for provoking a lot of pain, especially in the shoulder and upper limb regions. The facet joints lie posterior and lateral to the vertebral body, and their role is to assist

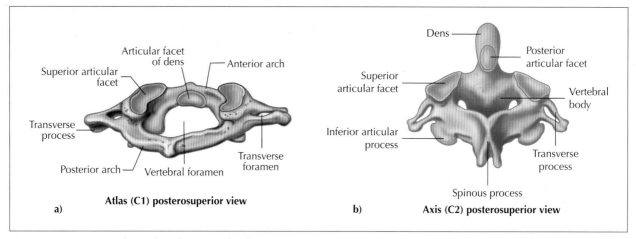

Figure 9.2: *Anatomy of: (a) the atlas (C1); (b) the axis (C2).*

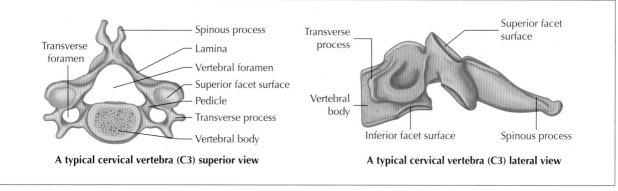

Figure 9.3: *A typical cervical vertebra from C3 to C7.*

the spine in performing movements such as flexion, extension, side bending, and rotation. Depending on their location and orientation, these joints will allow certain types of motion but restrict others: for example, rotation is freely permitted (cervical spine), but there is less range in lateral flexion.

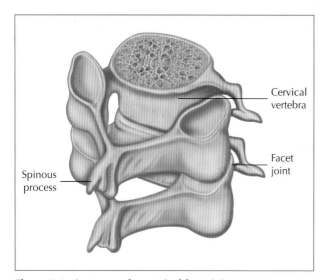

Figure 9.4: *Anatomy of a cervical facet joint.*

Each individual vertebra has two facet joints: the superior articular facet, which faces upward and works similarly to a hinge, and the inferior articular facet located below it. The C4 inferior facet joint, for example, articulates with the C5 superior facet joint.

Like all other synovial joints in the body, each facet joint is surrounded by a capsule of connective tissue and produces synovial fluid to nourish and lubricate the joint. The surfaces of the joint are coated with cartilage, which helps each joint to move (articulate) smoothly. The facet joint is highly innervated with pain receptors, making it susceptible to producing neck, shoulder, and even arm pain.

Motion of the Cervical Spine

This book is naturally about the nerves, and this chapter covers the cervical spine and its relationship to the exiting nerve roots. It makes sense therefore to include motion of the cervical spine as well into this chapter, because one has to consider the possibility that the cervical region is

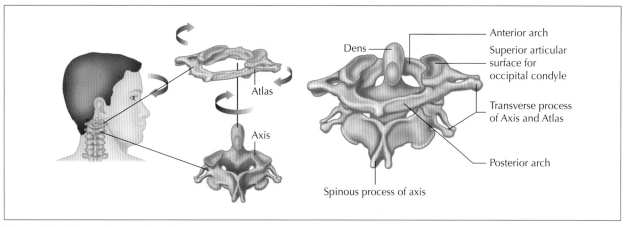

Figure 9.5: *Atlas motion on the axis.*

the source and potential cause of the patients' presenting symptoms.

The cervical spine is capable of motion in all three axes/planes of movement, allowing flexion/extension in the sagittal plane, side bending in the frontal plane, and rotation in the transverse plane. Circumduction is also possible as a gross movement, because of the summation of the other movements, although it is not recommended. The above-mentioned movements are represented throughout the cervical spine, but only because of the specific shape of the facet joints, which assist in guiding the movements for the specific spinal cervical segments, and which provide different emphasis of motion at different levels.

Motion of the Atlas (C1) and Axis (C2)

It is considered that the first 50% of the rotation (either left or right) of the cervical spine is mainly due to the atlas rotating on the axis, because this is a pivotal joint (Figure 9.5). In other words, if we take the normal range of motion (ROM) for cervical rotation to be approximately 80 degrees, then 40 degrees of that movement will occur between the levels C1 and C2.

Neurological Anatomy

There are eight cervical nerves that exit the cervical spine: the C1–4 nerves exit through the cervical plexus (see Figure 9.6),

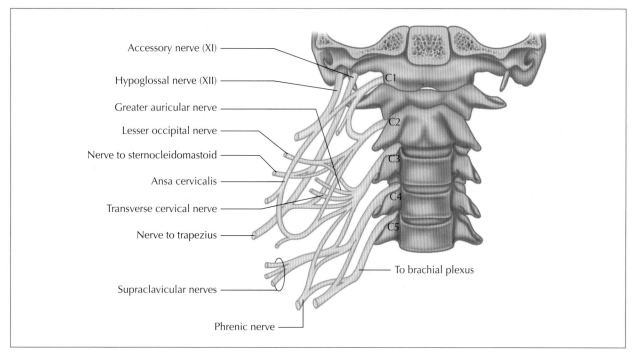

Figure 9.6: *Anatomy of the cervical plexus and the levels of the exiting nerve roots.*

and C5–T1 exit through the brachial plexus (Figure 3.4). However, there are only seven cervical vertebrae.

The first to the seventh cervical nerves exit *above* the level of the corresponding cervical vertebra C1–7 (Figure 9.6)—i.e., the C1 nerve exits above the level of the C1 vertebra, and so on. On the other hand, the eighth cervical nerve exits *below* the seventh cervical vertebra and *above* the first thoracic vertebra (i.e., the C8 nerve exits between C7 and T1).

The first thoracic nerve (T1 nerve root) then exits below the first thoracic vertebra (i.e., the T1 nerve root exits between T1 and T2). If you have a disc condition between, for example, C5 and C6, then the exiting nerve root of C6 could be contacted as a result of the disc problem. However, in the lumbar spine, if a disc condition is present at the levels L4 and L5, the L4 nerve root may be affected because it exits at the level below (as compared to nerve roots exiting at the level *above* in the cervical spine).

CASE STUDY 9.1

The first surgery I ever watched was an anterior cervical discectomy, which basically entailed the removal and subsequent artificial replacement of two of the cervical discs. This operation was performed on a 55-year-old female who had a few different and rather vague presenting symptoms. The more obvious symptoms she initially mentioned were pain localized to the left side of her cervical spine, and a radiating type of pain in her left shoulder and arm, with some inherent weakness during certain movements and in particular shoulder abduction.

This was confirmed as a posterior lateral disc herniation at the level C4/5 with contact to her exiting left C5 nerve root; the corresponding reflex was reduced, as was her myotome to that specific level. The latter is relatively simple and straightforward to diagnose in one respect, however, because she also had something going on that was bit more complex, namely a *central* disc bulge at the level C5/6 that was pressing on her actual spinal cord. This was a different story altogether, as she had various symptoms that she found difficult to explain. Her main complaint was that her left leg felt like it did not belong to her, and that she found it difficult to send the necessary information to her leg to get it moving.

When I watched the neurosurgeon perform the reflexes on her using the reflex hammer on her upper and lower limbs, all of them, apart from C5 (as the central disc was below this level), tested as positive and they were all increased; this is called *hyperreflexia* and classified as

3+++. The Babinski reflex was also positive (up-going plantar reflex), which indicates an upper motor neuron lesion of the CNS located in either the spinal cord or the brain. In this case, however, we knew her condition was from the spinal cord level of approximately C6.

The surgeon carried out the disc surgery (discectomy) to the levels C4/5 and C5/6, and replaced the discs with two artificial ones. The patient subsequently made a full recovery. A few weeks later at the follow-up appointment, the patient reported no more neck or arm pain, and more importantly regained the ability to control her left leg, with the reflexes (when tested) settling down to normal (2++); the Babinski reflex also tested normal.

As highlighted by Case Study 9.1, it goes without saying that the nervous system has a direct relationship to all the unique components that make up the cervical spine (CSP) as well as a relationship to the rest of the body. There are probably thousands of people throughout the world who consider their presenting upper limb (e.g., shoulder or arm) pain to be actually coming from the shoulder joint or the associated structures. For the majority, however, it may actually be the cervical spine and its associated exiting nerve routes that is the underlying causative factor of not only their presenting shoulder pain but also other symptoms they might have, especially if the symptoms are felt in the arm, hand, and fingers.

My own thought process is that the nerves, cervical spine, and even the shoulder joint are like a triangle or a three-way conjoined partnership. In the past, when I used to climb high alpine mountains, we would be roped together in a group of a minimum of three people for traveling safely across the snow. Simply put, if one part of the triangle (team) breaks down or becomes dysfunctional (or perhaps pathological in this case, as this is a medical relationship), then the other components will not be able to cope as easily and will have to compensate in one way or another. I always teach the following principle: if one has a problem with the shoulder complex, then eventually this becomes a problem with the cervical spine, and subsequently this has a knock-on effect on the exiting nerve roots; conversely, a problem with the cervical spine eventually becomes a problem with the spinal nerves, and subsequently this affects the shoulder and arm. The latter of these two concepts probably makes more sense to me.

I would like to share an interesting story with you. During a soft-tissue course, I asked whether anyone attending had shoulder pain, since that was going to be the next topic we would cover. Within a microsecond, a gentleman shot his hand up in the air and waved his arm vigorously at me from the back of the class, declaring "Yes, I have a *big* problem with my shoulder" (while keeping his arm in the air!). I responded by saying the following to the attendee: "I doubt that the arm which is currently still in the air is the painful arm, especially given the speed you lifted it." "Yes," said the man, "it *is* that arm which has the pain." There lies the problem, because to him, it was a *big* problem with his shoulder. However, I personally would classify it as a *little* problem with his shoulder, especially after the assessment and treatment, since it was not actually his shoulder that was the causative factor of his pain. You can probably guess that, given the nature of this text, the symptoms he felt around his shoulder were in fact referred pain, which was radiating from his cervical spinal nerves.

CASE STUDY 9.2

A local personal trainer friend of mine, who runs a cross-fit gym, referred one of his clients to me because they had difficulty performing one of the exercises in his routine. The exercise in question was to simply lie on the back on a bench and then extend the elbows using two dumbbells, as shown in Figure 9.7. This exercise is designed to strengthen the triceps muscle. You can see from the image that the left arm is unable to extend as far as the right one, and the reason for this is muscle weakness.

What I found interesting, however, was that the patient in question did not mention that he had any form of pain or even restriction in the neck, shoulder, and arms; he simply had a weakness in performing that particular maneuver. The personal trainer took a video of him performing the motion, so that I could gain a better understanding of the underlying problem. (I actually show this video to students on the neurological and cervical spine courses and ask them what they think the problem is and where the cause of the problem might be located.)

Some of you reading this will know straightaway what the problem was, but the majority will probably struggle, especially because he presented with no pain, restriction, or any type of obvious symptoms.

In earlier chapters I discussed power testing of the upper and lower limbs and referred to this as *myotome testing*. If you remember, I discussed watching a Canadian chiropractor who traveled over to the UK on an international lecturing tour and he kindly came to the clinic to treat a few of the Oxford University rowers, who were previous Olympians from Canada. Initially, he tests the power (myotomes) of the upper and lower limbs, and

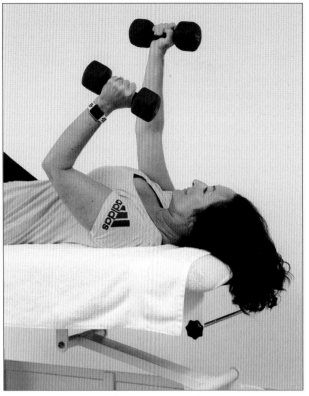

Figure 9.7: *Elbow extension exercise to train the triceps—the left side is limited because of muscle weakness.*

when he feels he has discovered a specific neurological weakness, he proceeds to adjust/manipulate the corresponding level of the spine. After the treatment, this chiropractor retests the power (myotome) of the motion, and hopefully this power then tests normal (grade 5).

I have been trying to use similar concepts ever since, so when I tested the above cross-fit patient and focused on the power of elbow extension, I found the left side to be very weak in comparison to the right side. If you look at the maps of myotomes in Chapter 7 (Tables 7.2 and 7.3), you will notice that the C7 myotome could have been a possibility for the level that was the underlying problem, as it mainly supplies elbow extension. However, the C7 myotome controls wrist flexion and finger extension as well, and when I assessed these two motions, they also tested weak for this patient. The C7 nerve root passes between the levels C6 and C7, so a disc condition was a possibility. However, because there was no altered sensation or pain, I considered that he had a rotated vertebra (or *subluxation* in chiropractic terms) that was tensioning the exiting C7 nerve, subsequently causing him weakness in extending his left elbow.

One of the analogies that I sometimes use is that of a dimmer switch. If you turn the switch in one direction, the light bulb becomes dimmer (less current is going to the bulb); if you turn it the other way, the bulb gets brighter (there is more current). If a nerve (wire) is being turned or compressed for some reason, say vertebral rotation, then the power (current) along the C7 nerve pathway will be reduced, and subsequently the movement or power of elbow extension provided by the triceps will show weakness (the bulb is less bright).

My treatment consisted mainly of a specific cervical spinal mobilization and then a manipulation technique to the left side of C6/7, upon which an audible cavitation was heard. I then retested the power of his left elbow extension and was very happy to find that the patient had regained normal power. The personal trainer messaged me a few days later to say that he had recommended training with his client and that there was no weakness present.

The reason I discuss Case Study 9.2 is to try to raise your awareness of an alternative way of assessing the upper limb through myotome testing of the neurological system. I know many therapists who consider pain in the shoulder complex, arm, and hands to *only* be originating from the cervical spine. This means that all the treatments they perform focus on the cervical spine and the exiting nerve pathways, rather than on the painful areas the patients are presenting with.

■ Cervical Spine Assessment

The physical therapist will need to ascertain if they consider the cervical spine to be involved in the neurological symptoms for a patient's presenting shoulder, arm, and hand pain. We could use what is known as the *KISS principle* (keep it simple stupid!), or the *keep it simple* principle: the patient is asked to perform the simple movements of rotation, flexion, extension, and side bending in order to see if these motions of the cervical spine exacerbate any of the presenting symptoms in the upper limb, which can include the chest, shoulder, axilla region, arm, hand, and fingers. If the symptoms in any of these areas are exacerbated by motion of the cervical spine, then one can realistically say that the cervical spine needs further investigation.

CASE STUDY 9.3

A 29-year-old female patient came to see me with pain in her left shoulder, with some referral to her left arm. The pain had only been present for a few days after the patient had suffered a bout of sneezing (it was "hay fever season").

The motion of coughing or sneezing (when asked) now exacerbated her symptoms and she was anxious about performing these simple actions because of the pain. Movement of her cervical spine to the left (rotation) also made her symptoms worse, as did bringing her chin down to her chest (flexion), especially when she was looking at her cell phone and replying to text messages.

On examination, I found the left C6 and C7 reflex to be 2++; however, the C5 reflex (biceps) on the left side was diminished, with a 1+ compared with the right side, where all the three reflexes were normal. The shoulder abduction and elbow flexion myotome (C5 myotome) was found to be a "3" on the test grading scale (a "5" is classified as *normal*). All other myotome levels were tested and had normal power. I performed light touch over the dermatome region of her upper limb and found she had altered sensation to the C5 dermatome.

I told the patient that I suspected she had prolapsed her disc at the level C4/5, and that the disc protrusion was contacting her exiting left C5 nerve root, which was responsible for her pain. I suggested an MRI scan to confirm the findings, which she had a few days later. I am pleased to say that, with weekly osteopathy treatment consisting of soft-tissue techniques and some gentle mobilizations and traction, the patient improved over the next few weeks to the point where the pain subsided, and she was discharged from the clinic.

I hope that reading Case Study 9.3 will convince you of the importance of cervical spine assessment as well as including the neurological examination using the reflex hammer and myotome/dermatome testing.

Active Range of Motion (AROM)

These tests are performed with the patient sitting on a couch.

Neck rotation:

- Instruct the patient to rotate their neck to the right as far as they comfortably can, and then to the left (Figure 9.8).
- Ask them to say if they feel any symptoms, restriction, or pain anywhere, and to focus in particular on their shoulder, arm, and hand.

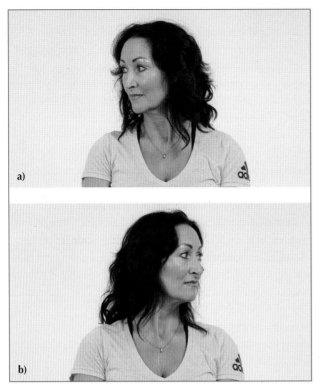

Figure 9.8: *AROM: neck rotation to the right (a), and to the left (b).*

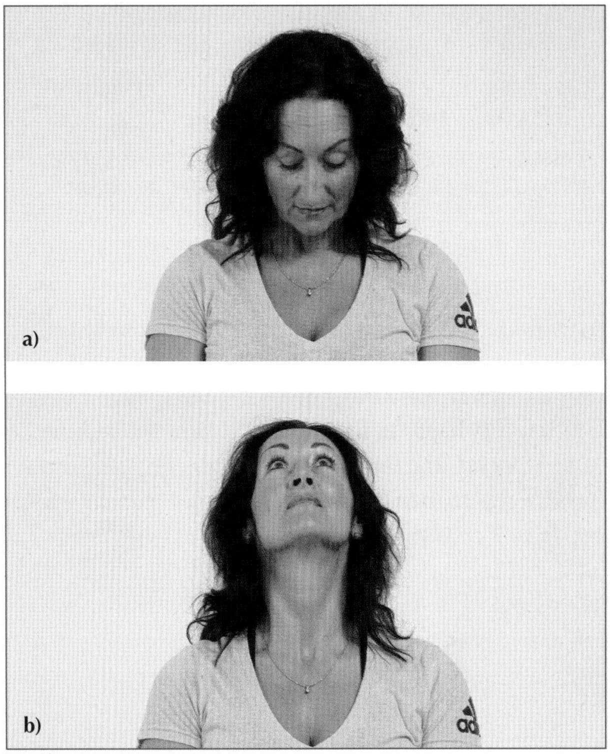

Figure 9.9: *AROM: neck flexion (a) and extension (b).*

Neck flexion/extension:

- Instruct the patient to slowly flex their neck by bringing their chin toward their chest, and then to slowly extend their neck by looking up toward the ceiling (Figure 9.9).
- Ask them to mention, as before, if they feel any symptoms.

Neck side bending:

- Instruct the patient to side bend (laterally flex) their neck by bringing their right ear down toward their right shoulder, and to repeat on the other side (Figure 9.10).
- Ask them to mention, as before, if they feel any symptoms.

Passive Range of Motion (PROM)

It is possible for all the AROM movements to be performed passively by the therapist with the patient seated; however, the movements are more commonly done with the patient in the supine position. Figure 9.11 shows two examples of passive movements—rotation and lateral flexion—although normally the entire cervical spine ROM would be tested passively.

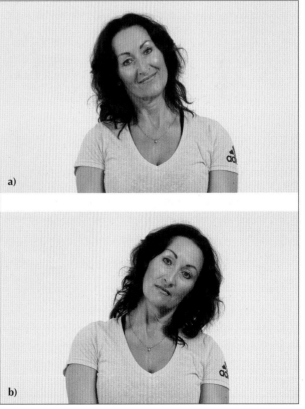

Figure 9.10: *AROM: neck side bending to the right (a) and to the left (b).*

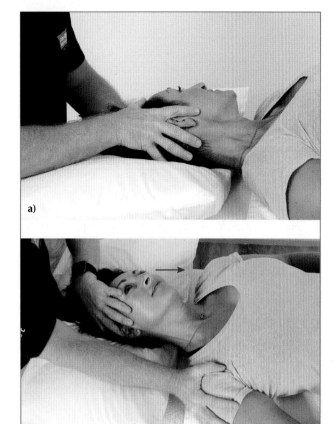

Figure 9.11: *PROM: cervical spine rotation (a) and lateral flexion (b).*

Note: If the patient has any pain or restriction in the active movements, but no pain/restriction when these movements are performed passively by the physical therapist, this usually indicates the soft tissues of the muscles and tendons are generally involved in the active motion. If, on the other hand, active movements *and* passive movements cause the patient's symptoms to increase, then one can assume that the cervical spinal joints are involved and will need further investigation.

Let me give you a couple of examples. The first example is of a 20-year-old patient who has strained one of their neck muscles, so that when they move their neck to the left and to the right, they are acutely aware of the pain. However, if I were to passively move their neck to the left and to the right, the movement would probably be almost pain free because the muscles should be relaxed (hopefully) during passive testing. Passive testing is used to assess the integrity of the joints and not generally used to test the integrity of the associated muscles.

My second example concerns a 65-year-old patient with a confirmed degenerative cervical spondylosis (osteoarthritis (OA)). When this patient moves their

neck to the left or to the right, it is very stiff, restrictive, and possibly painful over certain ranges. If I were to passively move this patient's neck to the right and to the left, I would also feel the restrictive motion, because of the underlying degenerative changes to the joints. Moreover, the patient would more than likely be aware of some discomfort during the passive motions.

Special Tests

There are numerous other specialized tests we can incorporate into our repertoire, some of which have already been covered earlier, such as reflex and myotome testing. We should therefore by now have a good idea whether or not the cervical spine is involved in the patient's presenting upper limb symptoms.

In terms of the cervical spine and special tests, I have already discussed and demonstrated what I would consider to be the best way of assessing this part of the vertebral column, and that is by means of the C5–7 reflexes, as well as individual power testing of the specific spinal myotomes and sensory testing through the dermatomes. However, there are also additional specific tests we can include to help with the overall diagnosis. Examples of the tests I might personally use in my clinic are given below.

Spurling's Compression Test—Cervical Nerve Root Pain

Spurling's compression test for cervical nerve root pain was first described by Spurling and Scoville in 1944, and Anekstein et al. in 2012 proposed a few variations of the procedure. It was suggested that a maneuver consisting of extension and lateral bending, which reproduced the patient's complaints in a tolerable fashion, be done first, followed by the addition of axial compression in the case of an inconclusive result.

- With the patient in a seated position, guide their head into extension and lateral flexion (Figure 9.12(a)).
- If there are no symptoms reproduced, gently apply a downward pressure to the top of the patient's head (Figure 9.12(b)).
- A positive sign is when the patient complains of pain that radiates into their shoulder or arm (dermatome).

Spurling's compression test

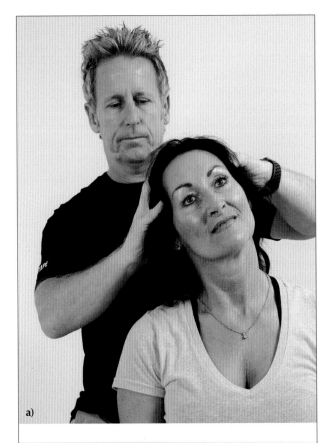

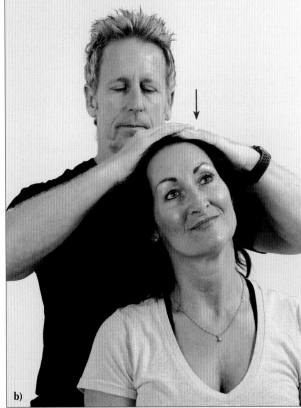

Figure 9.12: *Spurling's compression test: (a) patient extends and side bends their neck to the right; (b) therapist applies a downward pressure on top of the patient's head.*

Valsalva Maneuver Test

The Valsalva maneuver test was named after Antonio Maria Valsalva, a physician who specialized in the human ear. The Valsalva maneuver is used, for example, in diving to equalize pressure within the middle ear for descent.

With regard to the cervical spine and the nerves, the Valsalva motion can increase spinal pressure, so any space-occupying lesion, such as a disc prolapse with subsequent neural pain, can be exacerbated through the increasing pressure.

- For the typical Valsalva maneuver, ask the patient to try to equalize the pressure within the ears by blowing out through pinched nostrils, as shown in Figure 9.13(a).
- Alternatively, ask the patient to either suck their thumb or blow out onto the thumb, as shown in Figure 9.13(b).

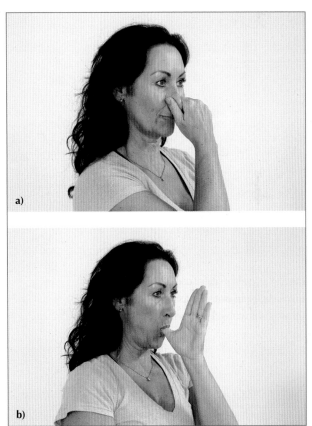

Figure 9.13: *Valsalva maneuver: (a) typical procedure; (b) alternative method involving sucking the thumb.*

Valsalva maneuver

■ Cervical Spine Conditions, Discs, Facet Joints, and Degeneration (OA)

It is believed that the majority of shoulder pain is directly or indirectly related to the cervical spine, and in this text, I would like to discuss some very common musculoskeletal structures that could be responsible for a patient's symptomology of pain perceived in the upper limb.

Disc Prolapse

The most common *disc disturbances*, as I like to call them, are: disc bulge, protrusion, extrusion, prolapse, herniation, and even sequestration (this is where the nucleus actually

detaches from the annulus). These variations of disc conditions are illustrated in Figure 9.14.

If we think back to earlier chapters, I discussed cervical spine conditions happening mainly at the disc levels C4/5, C5/6, and C6/7. Remember, there is no such thing as an actual slipped disc, even though it is often alluded to. It is the inner fluid, called the *nucleus pulposus* (located within the outer shell called the *annulus fibrosus*), that is generally responsible for the pain. This sensation of pain is only perceived when a pain-sensitive structure is contacted (e.g., posterior longitudinal ligament or exiting nerve root), which can refer the pain to the specific dermatome region (Figure 9.15). Think of my analogy of a tube of toothpaste— if you squeeze one end of the tube, the other end tends to bulge; the paste (nucleus) is pushing against the outer shell covering (annulus) from the inside, causing it to change shape, but there is no actual "slippage" of the tube.

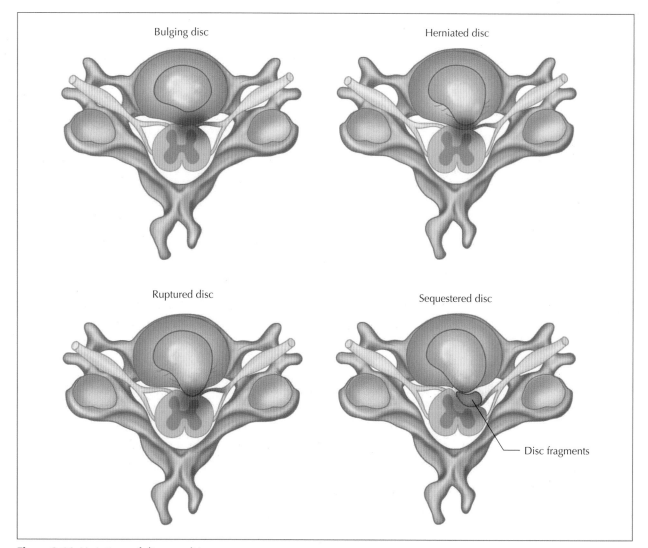

Figure 9.14: *Variations of disc conditions.*

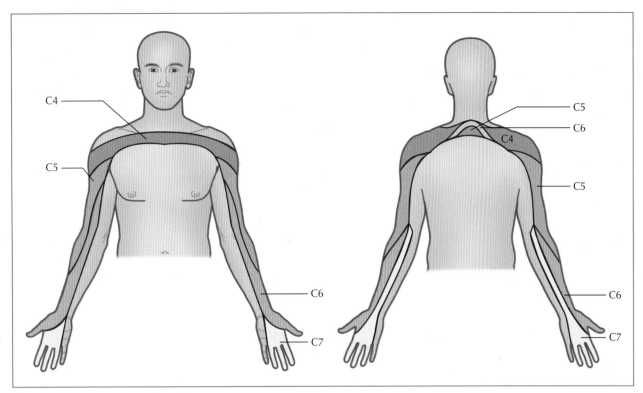

Figure 9.15: *C4, C5, C6, and C7 dermatome pain pattern.*

CASE STUDY 9.4

This is an interesting case of a 40-year-old lady who attended my clinic with her right arm held in the air and her hand down the middle of her back. I have seen this many times in the past, so I basically already considered a hypothesis of which structure was responsible for her pain. I said to her that the position she had adopted was probably the most comfortable position for reducing the pain in her shoulder and arm, and she categorically agreed! The patient then sat down and explained that she was worried because there was also pain in her right axilla and into her breast region; she thought that her breast tissue might be responsible and was panicking that it might be something nasty (cancer). I assured her that it probably would not be anything sinister, and I told her that I believed the symptoms she was experiencing were due to a compressed nerve in her neck, and that I considered it was originating from a cervical disc condition.

The pain had only been present for about a week, as her symptoms appeared after a ride at an amusement park and she felt her neck was "jolted" on a particular activity (dodgems). When she woke up the next day, the pain started to increase, especially in her neck, shoulder, axilla, arm, and even the central dorsal (top) aspect of her hand. When the patient brought her arm back to the side, the pain would intensify, so she would quickly put it back in the air and place her hand down her back. She said she did not know what else to do, as the pain was so excruciating.

For this patient, I kept the examination fairly simple (because of her pain), and found that the right C7 reflex was reduced (1+), and even on the verge of being absent (–), as compared to the C5 and C6 reflexes (2++). When I tested the C7 myotome, relating to elbow extension, wrist flexion, and finger extension, I found her to be very weak (Grade 1/2 out of a normal 5). I told her that I thought she had a disc prolapse between the levels C6 and C7, and that the disc was pressing on her exiting C7 nerve root, which was why she was experiencing her presenting symptoms. For some reason, I had a gut instinct that I needed another opinion before I treated her, so we arranged a scan. She saw a friend and colleague of mine for an initial consultation; he is a neurosurgeon and, surprisingly, he decided to operate all within one week of me seeing her. The surgeon simply said to me that it was probably the worst disc prolapse he had ever seen, and that she needed his help to remove the disc rather than see me for osteopathy treatment.

Case Study 9.4 demonstrates how essential it is to know when to refer someone on, as disc prolapses are very common in one respect, and thankfully they normally settle down over a few weeks. Typically, they can even be asymptomatic a lot of the time, so although a patient might have a disc condition confirmed by an MRI scan, it can generally be symptom free. It is the *rare* cases of disc pathology, however, that physical therapists may come into contact with that demand further investigation.

Cervical Spine Facet Joint

Cervical spine facet joints are highly sensitive structures and neurologically innervated through pain receptors (nociceptors)—so much so, that the facets have a high likelihood of causing debilitating and ongoing chronic neck, shoulder, and arm pain for thousands of patients.

Many of my previous patients have had cervical facet joint injections (guided through ultrasound) in spinal pain clinics throughout the UK before they come to me. They had the injections as a sort of diagnosis and a natural part of the treatment protocol to ascertain if these facet joints were responsible or partly responsible for their shoulder pain. In one respect, especially for the surgeon preforming the injection procedure, it is considered a major part of the diagnostic procedure, even though its use as a corrective treatment protocol is debatable. However, on a positive note, if the patient does have a reduction in symptoms in their shoulder after the injection, then the doctor can confirm a facet joint to be the possible causative factor. In my view, however, the whole musculoskeletal issue has been overlooked; this brings to mind the saying by Dr. Ida Rolf—"Where the pain is, the problem is not." I consider that these cases, where the patient has ongoing neck and shoulder pain, are likely to be the result of lots of small musculoskeletal manifestations that have caused long-term dysfunctional changes over the preceding years. And now the small inconsequential changes have slowly revealed themselves and become a larger problem, subsequently causing ongoing chronic pain for the patient.

Here is another analogy that might be applicable to these and other patients. I put forward that everyone has a "reservoir of compensation"; for some people, this is the size of a huge lake and will never run out of water, which is analogous to the body always being able to compensate, no matter what the problem. You will no doubt know friends and athletes like this who can participate in every sport, do all their daily tasks, and never complain of pain anywhere. For the majority of patients, however, the lake is a lot smaller and slowly starting to dry up, so now the body is struggling to compensate, which could explain their presenting symptoms. For example, a friend of yours has been a runner for 20 years, running three times a week every week, and suddenly in the last two months says that they are beginning to get pain in their lower back, knee, hip, foot (it does not really matter which body part hurts). Why? Because maybe, just maybe, their reservoir of compensation is starting to dry up.

Facet Joint Syndrome/Disease

Facet joints have a tendency to slide over each other, so they are in natural constant motion with the spine; like all types of weight-bearing joint, they can simply wear out and start to degenerate over time. When facet joints become irritated (the cartilage can even tear), this will cause the bone of the joint underneath the facet joint to start producing *osteophytes*, leading to *facet joint hypertrophy*, which is the precursor of *facet joint syndrome/disease* (Figure 9.16). This eventually leads to a condition called *spondylosis*, which is basically *osteoarthritis* (OA) of the spine—a type of syndrome or disease process that is very common in many older patients presenting with ongoing chronic neck and shoulder pain.

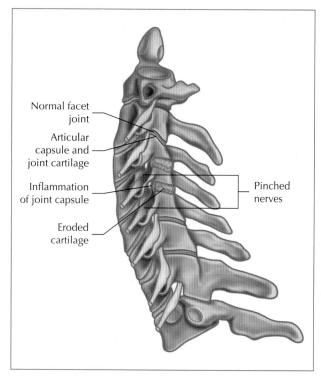

Figure 9.16: *Cervical spine facet joint syndrome/disease.*

CASE STUDY 9.5

A patient came into my clinic rubbing his right forearm and saying it was painful and had been for many weeks. He could not recall any specific incident relating to when or why this pain came on, but he did notice something was not quite right after a business trip away, when he stayed at a hotel for two nights. He found it very difficult to fall asleep in this hotel and felt that this was because of the different mattress and pillows as well as the large amount of noise from the road outside. He was told by his doctor that he had tendonitis in one of the wrist tendons in his arm, and was recommended to have a steroid injection, which he rejected, as he did not feel that this was the case.

On examination, I thought it would make sense to have a look at his arm just to make sure, and, as expected, I did not find anything particularly wrong—no tendinopathy present, as suggested by the doctor, although there was some slight tenderness in his forearm on palpation. Movements and testing of the elbow and shoulder joint also proved negative, so I then decided to focus on the cervical spine. I asked the patient to rotate his neck to the left, and it was no problem; however, when the patient rotated his neck to the right, the symptoms in his forearm increased. Next, I asked him to look over his right shoulder (a type of Spurling's test, which will be discussed later), and this motion again increased the symptoms in his arm. The reflex test results for C5/6/7 were 2++, and also the myotome tested strong for all cervical levels. I therefore concluded that either the C5/6 facet was inflamed and subsequently referring to his right arm, or there was some inflammation within the intervertebral foramen that was affecting the exiting C6 nerve root.

I proceeded to administer soft-tissue techniques to the muscles of the upper trapezius and levator scapulae, and then performed a mobilization technique, followed by a manipulative technique on the region of the C5/6 facet joint. The patient felt an immediate relief and has been pain free ever since, resulting in him being discharged from the clinic.

Cervical Spine Spondylosis (OA)

Unfortunately, this can occur sooner for some than others. The process of aging comes with some naturally degenerative changes, and certain areas of the human body, such as the hip and knee, can especially suffer. This holds

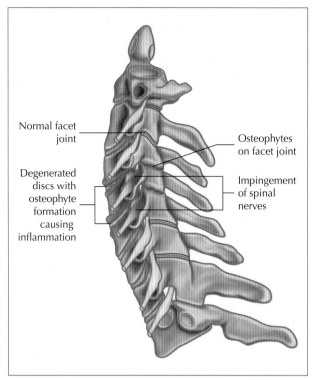

Figure 9.17: *Spondylosis (OA) of the cervical spine.*

true also for the lower three components of the cervical spine (C4/5, C5/6, and C6/7), as these areas can also become degenerative; in the spine, we call it *spondylosis* (*spondy* relates to "spine," and *osis* relates to "degeneration"). Spondylosis generally affects the vertebral bodies as well as the facet joints (Figure 9.17). The spaces through which the nerves exit, called the *intervertebral (neural) foramina*, can eventually narrow as a result of the underlying condition, causing painful neurological symptoms.

CASE STUDY 9.6

A 72-year-old female came to the clinic with generalized aching in both her shoulders, especially in the morning when she woke up. This ache would settle down after about 20 minutes, and she found some relief in having a hot bath or shower, which would reduce some of her symptoms. Her active range of cervical rotation was limited, especially to the left, and she kept saying that her neck "just felt stiff all the time."

When I performed passive rotation on her cervical spine in a supine position, her motion was still very restricted and uncomfortable. Surprisingly, the deep tendon reflexes and (myotome) power all tested normal. Her trapezius muscles felt exquisitely tender and very rigid on palpation, but she felt that a good massage would be of benefit. I said to her that I considered she had degenerative changes, and two weeks later an MRI proved that she had multilevel disc dehydration and degeneration of the vertebral bodies and facet joints, with osteophytic changes (bony spurs), especially to the lower three bodies of the cervical spine.

With regard to a treatment strategy, the patient asked me if I was going to manipulate her neck (using a high-velocity thrust technique, or HVT) and I replied that, under the circumstances, and especially since there were bony spurs and multilevel degenerative changes present, these techniques would not be appropriate and potentially could even be very dangerous. I said that soft-tissue techniques, gentle mobilizations, and muscle energy techniques to correct some of the shortened muscular tissues, along with some postural re-education exercises, would be my recommendations.

I told the patient that I would never be able to *fix* her neck, because of what was brought to light on the MRI scan; however, I did say to her that I would be able to *help* her in terms of improving some of her mobility and pain relief through soft-tissue techniques and gentle mobilizations.

■ Conclusion

The idea of discussing the anatomy, function, and basic assessment of the cervical spine was to make the reader aware of conditions that can exist within this part of the vertebral column and how they can affect the relationship to the exiting nerve roots. Remember, if any motion of the cervical spine, performed actively by yourself or passively by a therapist, as well as any of the special testing procedures, exacerbates symptoms anywhere in the patient's body, then realistically the cervical spine and subsequently the nervous system are involved and this requires further investigation.

10

Common Neuropathies Associated with the Nervous System

In reality, there are numerous medical books available to buy that relate to neuropathies. However, in this text my plan is to cover some of the most common neurological conditions affecting primarily the peripheral nervous system that the physical therapist might encounter in their own clinic. I mentioned at the beginning of this book that the focus would be mainly on the PNS, so the majority of all of the conditions I will discuss will be related to the exiting spinal nerves from the lower motor neuron (LMN), rather than on the CNS and specific conditions affecting the upper motor neuron (UMN). Neurological diseases that affect the UMN system—such as motor neuron disease (MND), multiple sclerosis (MS), and Parkinson's disease (PD)—are only covered briefly in this book (just MS and PD were mentioned in Chapter 5), because there are many texts and articles available for these specific conditions.

■ Peripheral Neuropathy

As mentioned above, the neurological conditions that will be discussed in this chapter are associated mainly with the PNS. If you were to do a Google search for "peripheral neuropathies," diabetes would be the most common type found by the search engine; it therefore makes sense to include this medical condition in this book. However, the complete list of all the possible peripheral neurological issues that can exist in the human being is not covered exclusively in this chapter. You will recall that, in previous chapters, many neuropathies have already been discussed, some through actual case studies. What is more, in the next chapter, on differential diagnosis, I will be discussing a multitude of other conditions for the neurological

system, as well as some of the underlying causative factors for a patient's presenting symptoms.

Typical symptoms of peripheral neuropathy are:

- Pins and needles, tingling, pain, or loss of sensation, perceived in the areas of the feet or hands
- A loss of balance or coordination, or an increase in weakness
- A cut or a lesion on the foot that does not heal

There are several variations of peripheral neuropathy and these are dependent on how many nerves are affected. A *mononeuropathy* will only affect one nerve—carpal tunnel syndrome is by far the most common example. If several nerves are affected, it is called *mononeuritis multiplex*, while if all of the nerves in the body are affected, it is called *polyneuropathy*. Polyneuropathy is one of the most common variations of peripheral neuropathy (e.g., diabetes), as typically the longest nerves are affected first, and the neuropathy generally starts in the feet.

There are four main classifications of peripheral neuropathy are:

- *Sensory neuropathy*, which can be affected by any trauma to the nerve that carries the sensory messages receptors (e.g., pain, touch, and temperature) toward the spinal cord and then to the brain. Typically, the symptoms are pins and needles, numbness, burning or sharp pain, and even loss of sensation regarding temperature or the inability to feel pain (this normally relates to the feet).

- *Motor neuropathy*, which affects the motor component and damage to these nerves will have an effect on the control of movement, so weakness or paralysis of the muscles is a possible sign (drop foot).
- *Autonomic neuropathy*, which, as the name suggests, means that damage to these specific nerves will affect the processes involved that occur involuntarily, and can cause problems with digestion (constipation or diarrhea), altered respiration rate, excessive sweating, rapid heart rate, and low blood pressure (which can make you feel faint, especially when you stand up).
- *Mononeuropathy*, which, as explained above, is damage to a single nerve (some of the neurological conditions presented below will be of this type).

In this chapter I am going to discuss the following neuropathies:

- Diabetes
- Bell's palsy
- Axillary nerve palsy
- Long thoracic nerve palsy
- Carpal tunnel syndrome
- Ulnar neuritis
- Radial nerve palsy
- Drop foot
- Thoracic outlet syndrome (TOS)

■ Diabetes

If I am truly honest, diabetes is something I do not personally see on a regular basis in my clinic, and this is mainly because of the age of my patients. Most of my clientele are students who are currently studying at the University of Oxford, and their ages range from 19 to 35; many of them are athletes and participate in a variety of sports, so the majority of these individuals are very fit and healthy.

What I would like to do now is to discuss the main effect of diabetes on the nervous system. Diabetes is the most common form of peripheral neuropathy and is classified as either *Type 1* or *Type 2*; it is commonly called *diabetic polyneuropathy* because it affects all of the nerves in the body, rather than just a single nerve (mononeuropathy). The main reason for this global effect on the nerves is the higher levels of sugar in the blood system when you have diabetes, which will eventually damage the small blood vessels that supply their associated nerves.

If you consider yourself to have a peripheral neuropathy that you think may be related to diabetes, then the diagnosis is relatively straightforward: the medical doctor will discuss your symptoms with you and will typically check the sugar levels in your blood and urine. The doctor might suggest a nerve conduction test with the neurologist to see how much potential damage has occurred.

Causes of Diabetes

Type 1 diabetes (insulin dependent) is caused by the inability of the body to produce enough insulin to regulate the sugar in the blood system; this results from the immune system attacking and destroying the beta cells of the pancreas, and there are currently no studies that show exactly why this process happens. The beta cells are the main types of cell located in the islets of Langerhans of the pancreas, and are responsible for producing and secreting the hormone insulin, which regulates the levels of glucose in the blood.

Type 2 diabetes (non-insulin dependent), on the other hand, happens when the beta cells from the pancreas are unable to produce enough of the hormone insulin, or when the body becomes resistant to this hormone, which is the most common reason for this condition. In general, the underlying factors for insulin resistance are the patient being excessively overweight and the general lack of regular exercise.

I was reading a statistic from Wikipedia saying that in 2017 there were over 425 million people in the world who have diabetes, with Type 2 making up 90% of the cases.

As regards the nervous system and the link to diabetes, there is no doubt that the condition can and will lead to a patient experiencing altered sensations; these symptoms typically start in both feet at the same time, and this is referred to as *diabetic neuropathy*. With both Type 1 and Type 2 diabetes, blood sugar levels become higher than normal, which is known as *hyperglycemia*. If the increase in blood sugar is not controlled, many complications will occur as a result of this, and neuropathy is ranked as the most common complication of this disorder. In numerous studies there have been lots of discussions about how the long axons are more vulnerable to damage as a result of the vascular supply to the peripheral nerves being naturally sparse, as there only a few arterioles (blood vessels) penetrating them.

The increased levels of sugar in the blood can eventually cause the blood supply to the peripheral nerve to be compromised and lack autoregulation, as demonstrated by Smith et al. (1977). This in turn makes the peripheral nerve prone to becoming ischemic (lack of blood to the tissues), which subsequently causes hypoxia (lack of oxygen) of the nerve itself, resulting in neuropathy. Dyck et al. (1984) proposed that microvascular injury is the most likely factor in focal nerve fiber loss of the distal axon in diabetes. Typically, the condition is described by patients as glove-stocking areas of numbness (in the hands and feet), as shown in Figure 10.1; the loss of sensation starts in the toes and feet and works its way backward to the ankle and lower leg, and later to the fingers and hands.

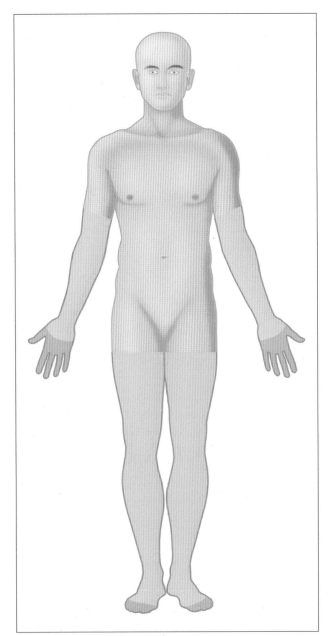

Figure 10.1: *Glove-stocking areas of altered sensory distribution in diabetic neuropathy.*

In diabetes, the nerve fibers in the epidermis of the skin are significantly affected, resulting in distortion and twisting with local swelling. The nerve fiber loss in the skin is associated with nerve fiber loss in the nerve trunk of the sural nerve, thus in keeping with the presence of clinically evident neuropathy, as discussed by Kennedy et al. (1986).

Sadly, as the condition progresses, patients lose the ability to feel pain in the balls of their feet; for example, they might not have the sensory feedback to know if they have stood on a splinter or on small, sharp stones on the beach. The overall likelihood of developing infections and ulceration therefore increases, which can eventually lead to gangrene and subsequent amputation.

CASE STUDY 10.1

I once saw a program on TV about medical accidents and emergencies, and one of the stories was about an older gentleman who was in the late stages of diabetes. He traveled with his family on holiday, and when sleeping in the bed on the first night, the man did not realize that the radiator had switched on and become very hot. Normally, this would not have been a problem, but in this case the radiator was actually in contact with the bed. During the night, the bed cover slid off, and one of his legs was then touching the radiator.

You can imagine what happened when he woke up in the morning and his family came into his room. Basically, the story continued, and it turned out that his leg had become physically stuck to the radiator and suffered serious burns; the emergency medical team had to remove his leg from the radiator. The prognosis for this man was poor: because of the inability of his body to heal from the sustained trauma, he ended up having his lower leg amputated.

Sensory Tests for Diabetes

In Figure 10.2 you can see a tuning fork being used to test the vibration of the lower limb. This might be one of the sensory tests one can do to ascertain if diabetes is present (as well as all of the other tests and initial consultation), because the sense of vibration is one of the first senses to be lost in diabetic neuropathy. Light touch and pin prick tests will indicate the sense of touch has also been affected.

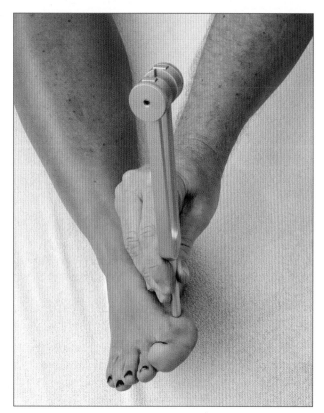

Figure 10.2: *Using a tuning fork to elicit vibration at the hallux.*

- Tap the fork to start it vibrating and initially place it on the sternum of the patient so that they can sense the vibration.
- Next, place the fork on the hallux and ask the patient if they feel the vibration and to say when they consider the vibration to have stopped.
- If the patient is aware of the vibration, that is a good sign. If they are not aware, then move the fork to the next bony landmark (e.g., the navicular tuberosity) and test again.
- Continue, if necessary, on to the next landmark (medial malleolus) and repeat, as this will indicate how much of the area is affected by the diabetes.

■ Bell's Palsy

Sir Charles Bell, a Scottish surgeon, first attributed the name Bell's palsy in 1929. There are no particular causes for this palsy condition (and is thus classified as *idiopathic*), and, generally speaking, it tends to resolve itself within three to four weeks (or thereabouts). As explained earlier, the condition is related to CN VII (facial nerve), which is called the *facial nerve*. Typically, the condition is associated with just a single nerve

(mononeuropathy), and the patient might exhibit the following signs and symptoms (see Figure 10.3):

- Inability to control the facial muscles on one side (e.g., raising the eyebrows or flaring the nostrils)
- Altered smile
- Impaired blinking and closing of the eyes
- Droopy eyelid
- Altered sense of hearing (sounds appear louder)
- Loss of sense of taste to the anterior two-thirds of the tongue (but only on the side affected by the palsy)

There is some evidence of a viral infection of CN VII in the facial canal of the middle ear in Bell's palsy.

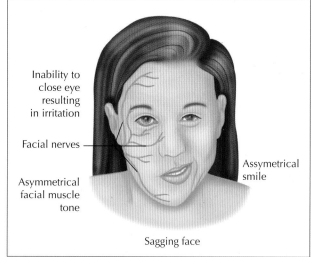

Figure 10.3: *Bell's palsy.*

CASE STUDY 10.2

Many years ago, one of the therapy students in my lecture during the nerve course I was teaching told me that she had had a brain tumor removed. As a result of the surgery there had been damage sustained to CN VII (facial nerve), and she now presented with Bell's palsy. It was such an interesting case that I thought I would share it with you.

The student in question said she could open her eyelid as normal, as this uses the levator palpebrae muscle, which is controlled by CN 111, the *oculomotor nerve*; however, she was not able to close her eye because of the weakness of the muscle responsible for that motion, namely the *orbicularis oculi*, which is controlled by CN V11. CN V11 of the person in this case study had been inadvertently cut during surgery to remove the brain tumor.

Amazingly, the medical team inserted a small gold weight in the patient's eyelid so that it could close under gravity—you could actually palpate this tiny weight! The lady said that, given the choice, she would prefer to have this condition (Bell's palsy) rather than the brain tumor, and that she was not particularly concerned that her condition would never recover because of the damage sustained to the facial nerve.

As I mentioned earlier, there are no obvious reasons why someone might get Bell's palsy, and if they happen to acquire the condition, it tends to resolve itself within a few weeks. The condition has been linked to diabetes, viral infections (herpes, influenza, and upper respiratory tract infections), pregnancy, migraines, and metabolic disorders, and is possibly activated by trauma and stress.

■ Axillary Nerve Palsy

This is an interesting one, as you might not see this condition very often unless you work, like myself, in a sporting context—for example, if you are the therapist for a local rugby team. If you happen to come across this condition, it is generally misdiagnosed by most physical therapists, and I will discuss the reason why. The axillary nerve originates from the C5 and C6 levels of the brachial plexus, exiting from part of the cervical spine. The nerve innervates the deltoid and teres minor muscles, as well as providing sensation to the "regimental badge" area (discussed in Chapter 3) of the shoulder region. When myotome testing (see Chapter 7) is performed, it would be relatively easy to see why the practitioner would suspect a C5 nerve root condition rather than an axillary nerve palsy, because the myotome for C5 is mainly from shoulder abduction of the glenohumeral joint, and we know that the deltoid muscle abducts the shoulder. However, if the therapist were to test the strength of the biceps through resisting elbow flexion (C5, C6 myotomes), the motion would prove to be strong (Grade 5), ruling out an actual C5 nerve root issue. Furthermore, the C5 reflex (biceps) would not be affected by damage to the axillary nerve.

Next, I would like to discuss two cases that I feel are of value when looking at this particular condition of the axillary nerve, as they might clarify what it is I am trying to put across to you. The first one, Case Study 10.3, is actually about me when I was in the military, while Case Study 10.4 concerns a patient who presented with what was considered by her medical doctor to be a sprained shoulder. The same diagnosis in Case Study 10.4 was also made by other practitioners who saw her, and they all mentioned the problem to be directly related to the shoulder joint, which was consequently the main focus of treatment by all of the therapists concerned. Would it not make sense, therefore, especially in the context of this book and the relationship to the nervous system, to cover all possible avenues, thus including the cervical spine as well as the shoulder complex in the equation?

CASE STUDY 10.3

When I was a physical trainer in the military, I organized a waterfall kayaking trip (my wild side) to North Wales with a few Royal Marine colleagues. The problem was that, at the time, I was by far the most experienced kayaker because I was qualified as an instructor and regularly participated in kayaking trips, whereas my colleagues were just starting out in this sport. When I discussed what I was planning to do over the weekend, they decided not to participate in the potentially more dangerous higher waterfalls, and I did not blame them for their decision.

I have personally kayaked these falls in the past, so I did not really see much of a problem. On the first day of the trip, we all started to kayak down the river, and all of us were able to safely make our way through all the white water, until we came to a set of three waterfalls (two of which were only just passable, while the third was very dangerous). My friends acted as the safety team, because I decided to kayak down these waterfalls on my own. For some reason, I took a different route from usual over the first fall, and had not noticed a large rock under the base of the waterfall. Subsequently, as I went over this fall with both arms in the air holding the paddle, I ended up contacting this rock with my right arm, and, because of the impact, I ended up capsized (basically upside down). The problem was, I was still stuck in the kayak with all the rushing water pounding on top of me, so I tried to perform an "Eskimo roll" (a technique used to roll the kayak back upright), because I knew the next waterfall was imminent. However, my right shoulder did not seem to allow the particular motion required for an Eskimo roll, so I pulled my spray deck off, releasing myself from the boat, and was now swimming. When I finally got to the edge of the river it became obvious that there was a problem with my arm; I suspected that I had fully dislocated my right shoulder, because of the unnatural position I could see my arm was in.

After being taken to hospital by ambulance and one hour later, an X-ray showed a full dislocation of my right shoulder joint. A few more hours later, I was put under a general anesthetic so that my shoulder could be relocated. The next morning when I woke up, the nurse was using a sharp object on the "regimental badge" area of my deltoid, and asked me if I could feel its sharpness. I said "No," and she responded that the nerve was probably damaged. At that time, I was not medically trained, so I was not sure what the nurse was telling me; the doctor elaborated, saying that it was the axillary nerve that was damaged, as that can be a complication of shoulder dislocations. He assured me, however, that the nerve would regenerate in approximately four to six months, and I am pleased to say that this was indeed the case for me.

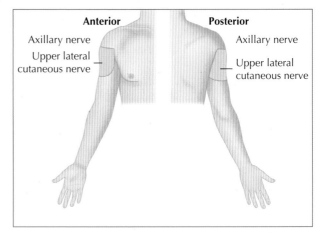

Figure 10.4: *Axillary nerve sensory innervation.*

CASE STUDY 10.4

A 28-year-old female likes to do yoga and meditation every morning as soon as she wakes up. Two weeks ago, after performing a movement called the *Down Dog* (a well-known yoga pose), she felt a sudden pain in her right shoulder and had to stop. She came to see me a few days later and was unable to fully abduct and flex her shoulder joint, mainly because of weakness rather than pain. Strangely, if the patient lay in a supine position (i.e., on her back), she was able to fully abduct, but not consecutively—she needed to rest for 30 seconds before she could lift her arm again. She also complained of a strange feeling at the deltoid insertion.

On examination, it was obvious that the deltoid muscle was unable to contract, and that other muscles, such as the pectorals and supraspinatus, were compensating. I told her that I suspected she had damaged the axillary nerve in her arm as a result of the yoga movement. This nerve is located close to the humeral head, and the patient was very mobile (even on the verge of being hypermobile); her humerus had been subjected to excessive motion because of her increased mobility, thus affecting the axillary nerve. I told her that the axillary nerve normally regenerates at a rate of 0.04″ (1mm) a day, so it would probably take her a few months to recover. The reason why she had felt a strange feeling in the deltoid area is the fact that the axillary nerve supplies sensation to the part of the arm known as the *regimental badge* (Figure 10.4), and if the nerve is damaged, altered neurological sensations will be perceived in that specific area.

■ Long Thoracic Nerve Palsy

The *long thoracic nerve* originates from the levels C5, C6, and C7, and innervates the serratus anterior muscle. This muscle is responsible for certain motions of the scapula, its main function being to protract and upwardly rotate the scapula (in combination with shoulder joint abduction); the muscle also maintains the scapula in suspension with the thoracic cage. If for some reason there is a weakness of this muscle, the scapula will probably take on a "winging" appearance.

CASE STUDY 10.5

I have suffered at some stage what I consider to be damage to my long thoracic nerve, even though I have not had any nerve-related conduction tests done to confirm the diagnosis. You can see from Figure 10.5 that my right scapula has excessive winging.

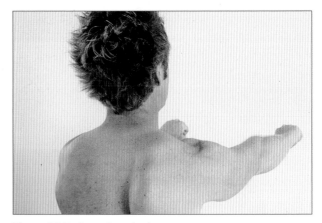

Figure 10.5: *Scapular winging.*

In my case, I reckon I have actually damaged my long thoracic nerve, rather than having a weakness of the serratus anterior muscle. I believe this happened when I went waterfall kayaking (see Case Study 10.3), took the wrong route off a rather high waterfall, hit a large rock below with my right arm, and dislocated my right shoulder. It was relocated under general anesthetic, and I woke up with damage to the axillary nerve. Unbeknown to me at the time, I probably sustained damage to the long thoracic nerve as well as the axillary nerve, likely due to the initial shoulder dislocation. However, jump forward 20+ years and I now have a permanent winging of the right scapula.

Over the years, I have tried to strengthen my serratus anterior muscle to try to help correct the winging and to promote correct stability to the scapula; however, if I am honest, nothing seems to have helped, and I am now resigned to the fact that perhaps this muscle might never regain its natural strength because of the nerve damage. I am generally happy with that because I do not have any pain and never really had any obvious symptoms in the first place.

As I mentioned earlier, I have never had nerve conduction tests, but if you look again at Figure 10.5 showing the scapula winging, I consider that I have permanent nerve damage to the *long thoracic nerve*. That is why I believe that all of the exercises I have done in the past to try to strengthen the serratus anterior have never really helped, because the underlying condition is related to a nerve and not a simple muscle weakness issue.

Remarkably, my shoulder never ever causes me a problem and I never suffer with any symptoms. To be honest, I quite like my "sticky-out" scapula—it is part of who I am, and I do not plan to change that. I actually like it, as it is my sort of party trick (even though I do not go to many parties these days!).

■ Carpal Tunnel Syndrome

I briefly mentioned carpal tunnel syndrome in Chapter 3 (brachial plexus), and the relationship of this condition to the median nerve. In terms of its definition, one could say that *carpal tunnel syndrome* (CTS) is a compression of the median nerve as it passes through the carpal tunnel. There are so many causes of carpal tunnel syndrome, and I remember once reading an article in which the author discussed some of these, ranging from something relatively simple (a lady who was pregnant and had swelling, or *edema*, in her arms) to something

rather complex (liver disease that subsequently caused an inflammation of the brain, or *encephalitis*).

If we look at the anatomy of the carpal tunnel a bit more, the space is formed between the four palpable bones of the hand, namely the trapezium, scaphoid, pisiform, and hamate. There are actually ten structures that pass through this small space: the four tendons of the flexor digitorum superficialis (FDS), the four tendons of the flexor digitorum profundus (FDP), the tendon of the flexor pollicis longus (FPL), and the median nerve, as shown in Figure 10.6. Any form of compression of the median nerve within the tunnel tends to cause pain, tingling, or numbness in the thumb, index finger, middle finger, and half (radial side) the ring finger (Figure 10.6).

In Chapter 3 I discussed the LOAF muscles of the thenar eminence and also how to test the strength of these muscles by means of the pinch grip (use the thumb to squeeze against the index finger), as this is one way of testing the activation of the median nerve. If the nerve is compressed within the carpal tunnel, the pinch grip will no doubt be weaker, and the thenar muscles of the hand might also start to atrophy (waste away). One can also use Phalen's test (or the reverse Phalen's test) to elicit the symptoms presented by the patient.

Phalen's Test

Phalen's test was first described by George S. Phalen, an American hand surgeon, for diagnosing carpal tunnel syndrome.

- Instruct the patient to flex their elbows and place the back of their wrists together.
- Ask them to hold this position for 30–60 seconds, to see if the presenting symptoms increase. This position induces compression of the tunnel (Figure 10.7(a)).

Reverse Phalen's Test

An alternative to the normal Phalen's test (and some texts actually consider this maneuver to be more effective) is the *reverse Phalen's test*. This test places the median nerve in a stretched position and also increases the pressure within the tunnel. The technique basically involves the opposite motion of that in Phalen's test.

- Instruct the patient to flex their elbows and place their palms together (extension of the wrist and fingers).
- Ask them to hold this position for 30–60 seconds, to see if the presenting symptoms increase (Figure 10.7(b)).

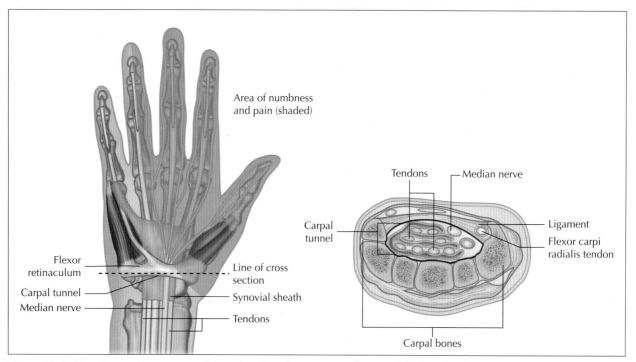

Figure 10.6: *Carpal tunnel anatomy and the related syndrome. Note: the use of finding the thenar eminence still sensitive is important (palmar cutaneous nerve of median preserved).*

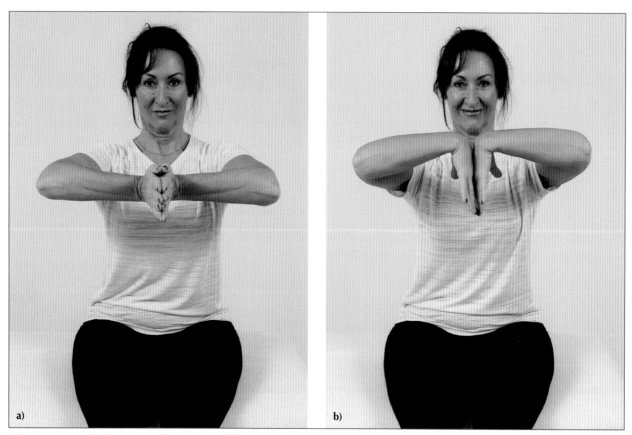

Figure 10.7: *(a) Phalen's test. (b) Reverse Phalen's test.*

Tinel's Sign

Another test that is frequently used to detect if a nerve is irritated is *Tinel's sign*, named after the French neurologist Jules Tinel.

- Lightly tap or percuss over the affected nerve, as shown in Figure 10.8.
- If the tapping increases the tingling in the affected areas of the thumb, index finger, middle finger, and half (radial side) of the ring finger, then this is a positive sign.

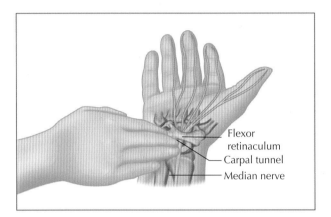

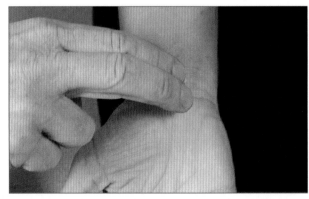

Figure 10.8: *Eliciting Tinel's sign by tapping the median nerve with two fingers. Tinel's sign is positive when lightly banging (percussing) over the nerve elicits a sensation of tingling, or 'pins and needles', in the distribution of the nerve.*

Tinel's sign is also commonly used to test the ulnar nerve within Guyon's canal of the hand (see below) or around the medial malleolus, as this nerve is exposed here and can be used for testing if the tibial nerve (from the sciatic nerve) is causing *tarsal tunnel syndrome*.

■ Ulnar Neuropathy

If you were to define *ulnar neuropathy*, potentially the patient might present with altered sensations in the areas of the little finger and half of the ring finger (ulnar side). The patient may also have difficulty with the use of their fingers (dexterity), and in severe cases might notice some atrophy of the muscles located within the hypothenar eminence. Again, like most neurological conditions, there are many causes.

This is an interesting one, because when I teach my students about this specific condition, I initially describe the nerve as originating from between the levels C7 and T1 of the cervical spine. This region of the spine is called the *cervical thoracic junction* (CTJ), and compression at this level can potentially cause associated symptoms in the hand. The nerve root that exits is referred to as the *C8 nerve root* and conjoins with the T1 nerve root to form the actual ulnar nerve. From the CTJ, the ulnar nerve then passes within the brachial plexus and through the thoracic outlet, so once again any compression at this level can exacerbate symptoms.

The main focus, however, is where the ulnar nerve passes through the cubital tunnel, which is formed by the medial epicondyle of the humerus and the olecranon process of the ulna. There is a condition called *cubital tunnel syndrome*, which signifies compression of the nerve in this particular area. The ulnar nerve is very susceptible to injury, as it is exposed just inside the medial epicondyle of the elbow; it is a known fact that the majority of ulnar neuropathies are caused here.

The nerve then proceeds into the forearm, passing into the wrist and continuing through the ulnar canal, termed *Guyon's canal*, as first described by French Surgeon Jean Casimir Felix in 1861. This is a tight tunnel in the hand, located between the pisiform carpal bone and the hook of hamate; the pisohamate ligament (roof of the canal) maintains these two bones together, as shown in Figure 10.9.

A condition known as *cyclists' palsy* affects the ulnar nerve and is sometimes caused by the unnatural hyperextended position of the hands on the handlebars. It tends to affect mainly long-distance cyclists, where the nerve at the level of Guyon's canal (or just slightly before) can become compressed and stretched.

As in the case of carpal tunnel syndrome, you can also perform Tinel's sign to elicit ulnar neuropathy.

- Lightly tap or percuss over the affected nerve near the medial epicondyle, as shown in Figure 10.10.
- If the tapping increases the tingling in the affected area of the little finger, then this is a positive sign.

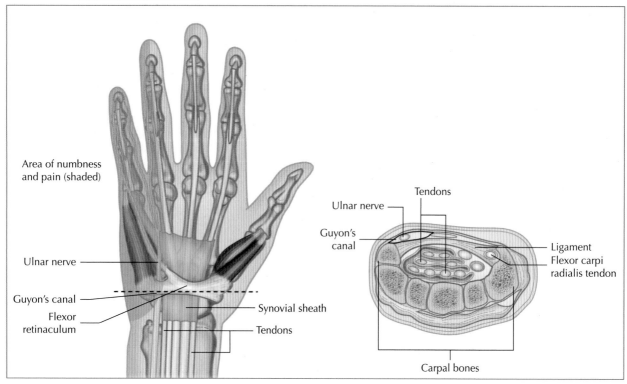

Figure 10.9: *Ulnar neuritis and Guyon's canal.*

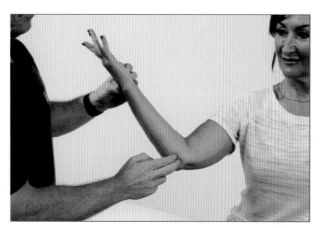

Figure 10.10: *Eliciting Tinel's sign by tapping the ulnar nerve near the medial epicondyle with two fingers.*

■ Radial Nerve Palsy

CASE STUDY 10.6

I would like to tell you about a fascinating case study regarding the radial nerve and a particular injury I had never seen before. Many years ago, while I was weight training in the gym, I met a mature student from the US who was studying for a master's degree at the University of Oxford. He knew I was medically trained, so one day he showed me a scar just above his elbow; he said when he was in Iraq during the conflict, he was shot and the bullet went through his body and passed through his liver and spleen, finally exiting through his elbow. Amazingly, he survived this trauma and naturally the life-threatening injuries were dealt with first and foremost; his arm was initially just patched up, and it was not until many months later that it was finally looked at.

The bullet had basically passed straight through his humerus bone and obliterated his radial nerve, and as a result of this injury he was left with a condition called *wrist drop* (limp wrist), as illustrated in Figure 10.11. If you recall from the discussion of the radial nerve sensory supply in Chapter 3, the radial nerve supplies all of the muscles that are responsible for extension of the elbow (triceps), as well as all of the wrist extensor muscles. Because the nerve was damaged above the elbow, the injury naturally only affected the muscles below the elbow, and so the action of the triceps and thus extension of the elbow was normal. However, it was very obvious that he did not have the ability to contract the muscles governing the specific motion of wrist extension.

The surgeons said it was probably a little too late to try to reconnect the two ends of the damaged radial nerve;

instead, they rerouted a flexor tendon of the forearm to the dorsal aspect of the wrist, so that it now became a sort of extensor muscle. The surgeons also shortened the wrist extensor retinaculum to form a kind of splint. Either way, what they did really helped this guy—he felt that he was not perfect in terms of function and strength, but, looking at him, you would never have known that he had a wrist weakness. Personally, I thought it was totally miraculous and inspiring just listening to his story, as I also spent time in Iraq during the conflict (I was a soldier in the British Army), although we were over there at different times.

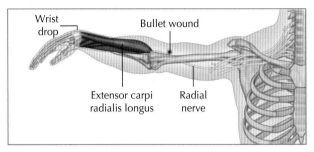

Figure 10.11: *Radial nerve palsy—wrist drop, caused by a bullet wound. The key muscle in respect to wrist drop is extensor carpi radialis longus.*

Miscellaneous Radial Nerve Damage

Some other types of damage to the radial nerve, which have been given unusual (but apt) names are *Saturday night palsy*, *honeymoon palsy*, and *crutch palsy*.

Saturday Night Palsy
During my time in the military, alcohol overuse seemed to be a natural and regular occurrence. When some soldiers drank more than they were capable of handling, they became intoxicated, and then had the ability to sleep anywhere. It is acknowledged that if one sleeps in a chair with an arm resting over the back, and stays in that position for several hours, there is a risk of potential damage to the radial nerve located in the axilla (armpit).

Honeymoon Palsy
If somebody else is sleeping on your arm for long periods (e.g., overnight), then this again can cause damage to the radial nerve.

Crutch Palsy
If you have ever fractured your leg, you will have probably been given a set of crutches to use. Crutch palsy, as you can probably guess, results from the use of axillary crutches, which are placed under the armpits to assist

in walking. However, the use of such crutches is not as widespread as in the past, which naturally means a reduction in the occurrence of this type of palsy.

■ Drop Foot

Drop foot can be defined as a significant weakness in ankle and toe dorsiflexion, as shown in Figure 10.12, and there are many causes of this condition, as I will discuss shortly.

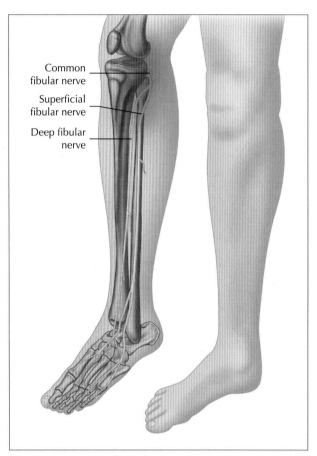

Figure 10.12: *Drop foot.*

The ankle and foot dorsiflexors include the tibialis anterior, extensor hallucis longus (EHL), and extensor digitorum longus (EDL) muscles. These muscles assist the body in extending (dorsiflexing) the ankle and foot, so that the leg clears the ground during the swing phase of the gait cycle, and they also stabilize the foot in preparation for the its initial contact with the ground (heel strike). Furthermore, these muscles control some of the pronation (flattening) of the ankle and foot by eccentrically contracting (lengthening while in a state of contraction) during the stance phase of the gait cycle.

Drop foot is also typically called *steppage gait*, or may even be referred to as *slap foot*, because the patient tends to walk with an exaggerated flexion of the hip and knee in order to prevent the toes from catching on the ground during the swing phase of the gait cycle. This, in turn, will cause the foot to naturally plantarflex, because the weak muscles are unable to control the dorsiflexion motion, and the foot will then potentially slap the ground.

Three specific case studies (10.7–10.9) have been chosen to highlight potential secondary consequences from a primary trauma. It is important to note how these three initial presentations are identical in one respect (all of the patients are unable to dorsiflex their ankle and foot) but vary widely in another (the underlying factors for the cause of the condition are completely different).

CASE STUDY 10.7

A 24-year-old male presents with an inability to dorsiflex his ankle.

Medical History
Six weeks before his initial consultation, this rugby player had gone in for a tackle and twisted his ankle while playing for his local team. At the time of the incident, he felt a sharp pain and heard a cracking sound. He was taken to the hospital's emergency department and given an X-ray, which showed a fracture of his tibia. A plaster of Paris (POP) cast was applied over his lower leg up to the knee, and he was told to return in a few weeks.

When the fracture healed after approximately six to eight weeks, the cast was removed, and the patient was advised to begin mobilization exercises to naturally encourage ROM through his ankle and foot. However, he found dorsiflexion very difficult to perform because of what he believed was weakness of the muscles; he thought this was normal because his leg had been in a cast for many weeks. Even though his ability to dorsiflex was extremely weak, to the point that there was hardly any movement, the action itself did not cause any pain. The nurse subsequently advised him that his muscles were weak and suggested he try physiotherapy. Rather than wait for an appointment on the UK's National Health Service (NHS), his mother booked an appointment for him at the sports injury clinic.

CASE STUDY 10.8

A 22-year-old male presents with an inability to dorsiflex his ankle.

Medical History
Two weeks before the consultation, this athlete had gone in for a tackle while playing football. He remembered being kicked on the side of the leg and said he felt an excruciating pain shooting down his anterior shin.

After this happened, he went to the side of the pitch and immediately iced the anterior part of his leg, because that was where he felt the symptoms; he also applied a compression bandage over the injured site. Ever since the injury occurred, this patient has been struggling to walk normally. He finds it difficult to lift his foot off the ground while walking, and describes his foot as "slapping" the ground on impact.

Discussion of Case Studies 10.7 and 10.8

Both of the athletes in these two case studies presented with exactly the same symptoms (i.e., they were unable to dorsiflex the ankle), so drop foot was the diagnosis.

When you come across situations like this, in which the main muscle involved in dorsiflexion (the tibialis anterior) is shown to be weak—or in more severe cases, unable to demonstrate a contraction—then the possibility of a problem with the nerve controlling the muscle needs to be considered. The nerve in question is the *deep fibular nerve*, which is a branch of the common fibular nerve. Fibers from the dorsal branches of L4–S1 are found in the common fibular nerve, which pairs with the tibial nerve to constitute the sciatic nerve (L4–S3). The sciatic nerve leaves the pelvic cavity at the greater sciatic foramen, just inferior to the piriformis muscle.

The sciatic nerve divides to form the common fibular and tibial nerves near the distal thigh, just above the popliteal fossa, as shown in Figure 10.13. The tibial nerve continues all the way down the posterior compartment of the leg and into the plantar surface of the foot. The common fibular nerve crosses laterally over the fibular neck to the anterior compartment of the lower leg, dividing into two separate

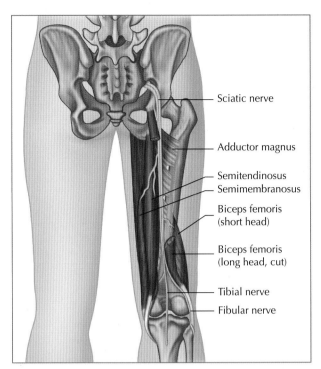

Figure 10.13: *The division of the sciatic nerve into the common fibular and tibial nerves.*

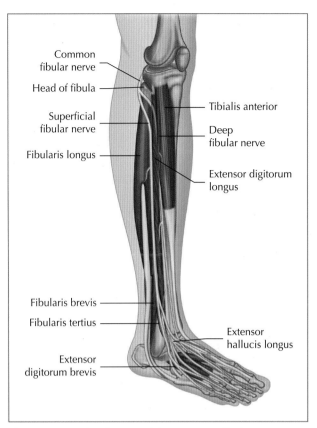

Figure 10.14: *The division of the common fibular nerve into the superficial and deep fibular nerves.*

branches called the *superficial fibular nerve* and the *deep fibular nerve* (Figure 10.14).

The superficial fibular nerve supplies the peronei muscles and then branches to the anterolateral area of the ankle to supply sensation to the dorsum (top) of the foot. The deep fibular nerve supplies the tibialis anterior, extensor hallucis longus, and extensor digitorum longus muscles, and also provides cutaneous sensation to the web space between the first and second digits.

The common fibular nerve is susceptible to injury all the way along its course, but is particularly vulnerable to trauma at the point where it passes around the neck of the fibula.

So, back to Case Studies 10.7 and 10.8. It was fairly obvious from Case Study 10.8 that the football player had sustained trauma to the deep fibular nerve because he was kicked on the side of his leg, which could quite easily have damaged the nerve in question.

Case Study 10.7, however, is a different story. Yes, the rugby player had suffered an injury—but this was to his ankle originally, with a subsequent fracture, so why did he have drop foot after the removal of the POP cast? Let's consider the clinical reason behind this; drop foot in this case was probably due to compression of the common

fibular nerve caused by the POP cast exerting pressure near to the neck of the fibula. Initially, there would be no obvious symptoms, but if you compress a nerve for many weeks then, of course, there will be consequences—in this case, drop foot.

CASE STUDY 10.9

A 45-year-old male presents with an inability to dorsiflex his ankle.

Medical History

This gentleman telephoned me a few months before he eventually came to see me for a consultation at the clinic. He told me that all the therapists he had seen in the past, as well as the doctor, said his drop foot problem originated from his lower back; in particular, disc pathology was mentioned as well as compression of the L5 nerve root. This all sounded pretty feasible; however, the patient never mentioned any symptoms of back pain or any significant injury he had sustained to his lumbar spine, and he thought the problem might be coming from another structure. I agreed and said that I did not believe his lower back was causing the symptoms. Anyway, a few months later he had an X-ray and MRI scan, but the images showed nothing of significance, and basically that there was no L4 or L5 nerve root compression, or any type of disc condition for that matter.

When I assessed his ability to dorsiflex, there was no obvious motion. I then asked him to try to lift (extend) his great toe (hallux), and again there was no activation of any of the associated muscles. I therefore decided to initially look at the head of the fibula and the attachment to the tibia, an area known as the *proximal tibiofibular joint*, which is classified as a *synovial gliding joint*. I wanted to see if there was any restriction present in this joint, since the common fibular nerve is in close proximity to the head of the fibula. I found this joint to be particularly stiff, and so I performed mobilization techniques to promote the mobility; I also used some soft-tissue techniques to the fibulares, tibialis anterior, and extensor muscles of the digits and hallux.

Remarkably, a few days later, the patient said he felt a slight improvement, so I decided to focus the treatment on mobilization of the tibiofibular joint and soft-tissue work to the muscles. Over the next few weeks and months, we saw some improvement, and I was pleased to see that around six months later, there was significant improvement in the activation of the tibialis anterior and extensor (EDL and EHL) muscles, to the point where I believed that drop foot was now absent, and I subsequently discharged the patient from the clinic. I believe that this patient improved relatively quickly because I was able to release the pressure off the deep fibular nerve, which then allowed it to regenerate.

Think back to Case Study 4.2 in Chapter 4—that patient also had drop foot, caused by his proximal tibiofibular joint. The difference in that case, however, was that an MRI showed a cyst located within the lateral compartment of his lower leg; the cyst was approximately 17″ (7cm) in length and 1″ (2cm) in width, and it had somehow encased part of the deep fibular nerve. The consultant radiologist postulated that this had resulted from a synovial fluid seepage from the tibiofibular joint. The reason why I believe the overall prognosis was poor (he still had drop foot, even after the surgery to remove the cyst around the deep fibular nerve) is because the problem had been present for over a year or two.

Common Fibular Nerve Treatment and Repair

After reading the causes of the conditions in Case Studies 10.7, 10.8, and 10.9, would you not think that a therapist would be very tempted to treat the area of weakness by at least trying to strengthen the muscles that were tested as weak? Remember, however, the underlying factor for these three cases is actually a neurological one, and the cause is not simply muscle weakness. Therefore, strength exercises in reality will not have much of an effect.

Research shows us that the common fibular nerve is able to regenerate by approximately 0.04″ (1mm) per day; research also shows that this does, however, depend on how long the nerve has been compressed. If nerve recovery takes longer than about a year, say, then the paralysis could actually be permanent; moreover, nerve injuries located more than a few inches from the muscle do not recover well. Surgery may be an option to correct or alleviate the underlying problem causing drop foot; for example, if drop foot is caused by nerve compression from a lumbar herniated disc, a spinal surgical procedure called *discectomy* (removal of part of the disc that is in contact with the nerve root) may be required in order to relieve the pressure.

CASE STUDY 10.10

I recently read a book called *Do No Harm*, written by the neurosurgeon Dr. Henry Marsh. In one chapter, I recall him talking to a patient about having a discectomy, because the patient was experiencing a lot of back and leg pain. He assured the patient that the procedure was relatively straightforward, but the problem was that a colleague of his performed the surgery instead. When Dr. Marsh went to check on the patient's progress, he noticed that the actual L5 nerve root had been cut by mistake. The patient now had to be told that he would have permanent drop foot for the rest of his life as a result of the mistake, because the L5 spinal nerve root could not be reattached and would not regenerate, as compared to the peripheral nerve, which typically has the ability to regenerate.

Other Possible Causes of Drop Foot

In clinical practice there are numerous presentations in which the client has obvious drop foot but the cause is not related to trauma. As not all clients participate in sport, you should be aware of conditions outside the scope of the sports medicine field, such as:

- Lumbar disc herniation affecting the L4 and L5 nerve roots
- Spondylolisthesis (slipping of a vertebra)
- Compartment syndrome
- Hip-replacement surgery
- Knee arthrotomy
- Acupuncture near the head of the fibula

Awareness is Key

Drop foot is not seen very often at the sports injury clinic, but when it does present itself, the first-line practitioner should have at least a basic understanding of the potential conditions that could be causing these signs and symptoms. The good thing is that the patients in Case Studies 10.7 and 10.8 made a complete recovery over a relatively short period of time, thanks to the nerve regeneration capability. In these two cases, rest was prescribed in order to let nature do what it does best—heal. The patient in Case Study 10.9, on the other hand, showed some improvement but the diagnosis of drop foot was still maintained, because I believe the condition was probably left for too long before surgical intervention.

In terms of self-help to prevent the muscles atrophying (or wasting), a TENS (transcutaneous electrical nerve stimulation) machine can sometimes help. This device causes the muscles to contract, thus preventing atrophy, and might even assist the nerve in its regeneration because of the electrical signals being sent through the muscles.

■ Thoracic Outlet Syndrome

The brachial plexus (C5–T1), subclavian artery, and returning subclavian vein, known collectively as the *neurovascular bundle*, exit at the root of the neck on their journey to the upper extremity, hand, and arm through a small space called the *thoracic outlet*, which lies between the collarbone and the first rib. The brachial plexus and subclavian artery pass through the natural space formed between the anterior and middle scalenes, called the *interscalene triangle* (Figure 10.15(a)). Note that the subclavian vein does not normally pass through this interscalene triangular space; instead, it passes adjacent to the anterior scalene muscle, and there is a natural groove formed over the first rib for the passage of the vein (Figure 10.15(b)).

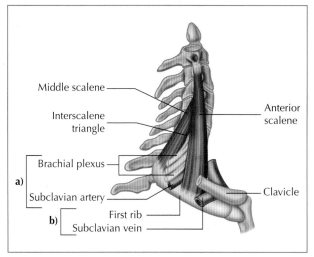

Figure 10.15: *(a) Passage of the brachial plexus and subclavian artery through the interscalene triangle. (b) The subclavian vein and its passage adjacent to the anterior scalene and over the groove in the first rib.*

These three structures now continue their journey (even though the vein is returning) and pass over the first rib and under the clavicle, as well as passing underneath the pectoralis minor, and there is no doubt that these delicate tissues can be compressed anywhere along the pathway. Because the structures are neural as well as vascular, the patient's symptoms can be anything from pain, numbness, tingling, paresthesia, or weakness to temperature changes and even swelling to the area of the shoulder, arm, forearm, hand, and fingers.

Many articles have been written about this subject matter; however, I feel this topic needs to be covered from another perspective, as the history of thoracic outlet syndrome (TOS) started back in 1861 when a 26-year-old female had a painful and ischemic left arm. The diagnosis of a cervical rib (which is an abnormal projection from the transverse process of the C7 vertebra) was made, even though there were no X-rays available at this time, and it was Mr. Holmes Coot who successfully performed the surgical excision of this extra forming rib.

There are three different types of TOS:

1. *Arterial*, caused by compression of the subclavian artery.
2. *Venous*, caused by compression of the subclavian vein.
3. *Neurological*, caused by compression of the brachial plexus.

Rob and Standeven in 1958 reported ten cases of arterial occlusion as a complication of what they termed *thoracic outlet compression syndrome* and thus introduced the term to the surgical literature.

According to Vanti et al. (2007), *nonspecific neurogenic TOS* makes up the bulk of diagnosed cases of TOS, as most patients have neurological symptoms. They suggest it may account for up to 85% of TOS cases and often follows an ulnar nerve (C8/T1) distribution.

Typically, the lower medial cord of the brachial plexus is affected, and the symptoms are generally related to the nerves from levels C8 and T1. The ulnar nerve originates from the roots of these two levels; also subdividing from these levels are the cutaneous (sensory to the skin) nerves, namely the medial brachial and medial antebrachial nerves. The C8 and T1 dermatome will affect mainly the medial aspect of the arm and forearm, the hypothenar eminence of the hand, the little finger, and half the area of the ring finger.

Compression of the subclavian artery (please note that this condition is very rare) is normally associated with a cervical rib or first rib anomaly causing a narrowing of the artery, with the potential to form an aneurysm just beyond the site of compression. The coldness to the hand and seemingly diminished blood supply (subclavian artery compression) could well be due to irritation of the sympathetics on the vessel as compared to narrowing of the subclavian artery itself. (See also the section on cervical rib.) The patient might perceive the following symptoms: a sudden onset of hand pain and weakness, arm fatigue with numbness, and tingling in the fingers. The fingers will feel cold and pale with diminished sensation, and the patient will remark that if any wounds are sustained to the arm and hands, they are very slow to heal. If compression of the subclavian artery is suspected, an immediate medical referral is recommended. A capillary refill test of the nail bed will indicate a low refill rate because of the slow blood flow to the nail. Alternatively, if Allen's test (tests the speed of blood flow to the hand—see below) is used, the result will be positive.

TOS—Special Tests

Allen's Test
Allen's test is performed with the patient seated.

- Passively lift the patient's arm and ask them to clench their fist quickly several times (3–5 times is normal). This maneuver will stop the blood flow to the hand (Figure 10.16(a)).

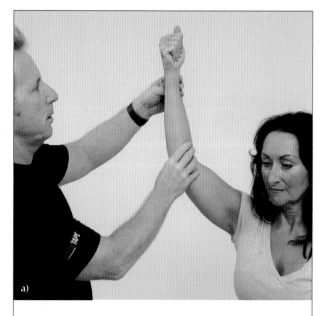

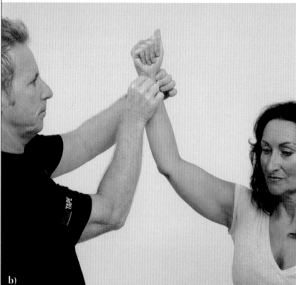

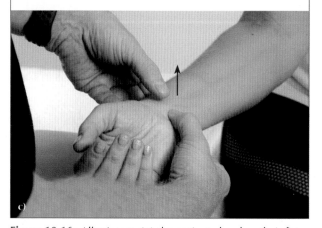

Figure 10.16: *Allen's test: (a) the patient clenches their fist 3–5 times; (b) the therapist compresses both the radial and ulnar arteries; (c) the radial artery is released and the time is noted for the blood to refill.*

- With the patient's fist still clenched, compress both the radial and ulnar arteries of their wrist (Figure 10.16(b)).
- Lower the patient's arm and ask them to open their fist while you still apply pressure to each of the arteries.
- First, release the radial artery (Figure 10.16(c)), and note the time it takes for the capillary refill.
- Repeat the whole procedure, but now release the ulnar artery and measure the capillary refill time.

Allen's test is designed as an arterial vascular test to rule out distal arterial disease in patients with symptoms of tingling and numbness in the hands. By compressing both distal arteries and pumping the fist, blood is effectively eliminated from the hand. Then, by releasing one artery, the hand perfusion time can be measured and compared with normal values, thus ascertaining the effectiveness of each artery. Allen's test has an important defect in that the blood in the superficial palmar arch (from the ulnar artery) is much nearer to the surface so is likely to "brighten up" quicker than the deep arch (radial artery).

Adson's Test

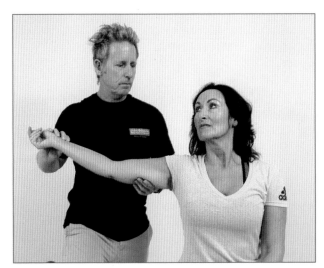

Figure 10.17: *The therapist externally rotates, abducts, and horizontally extends the patient's shoulder, and the patient takes a breath in, while the pulse is being monitored.*

Adson's test is performed with the patient seated.

- Locate the radial pulse in the patient's symptomatic arm.
- Ask the patient to rotate their head *toward* the affected side and to extend their head and neck back.
- Externally rotate the patient's shoulder, abduct it to 90 degrees, and horizontally extend it to 10 degrees.

- From this position, ask the patient to take a deep breath and hold it, as shown in Figure 10.17, while you continue to monitor their pulse.
- Ask the patient to say if they feel any changes in their arms or hands.

Adson's test increases tension in the scalene muscles, potentially compressing the neurovascular bundle. Gillard et al. (2001) reported that Adson's method was one of the better performing tests among those commonly used for TOS, having a positive predictive value of 85%. In that particular study, either a loss of the radial pulse or a reproduction of symptoms was considered to be positive. A positive Adson's test suggests that the scalene muscles should be assessed and treated for hypertonicity and trigger points.

Roos Test

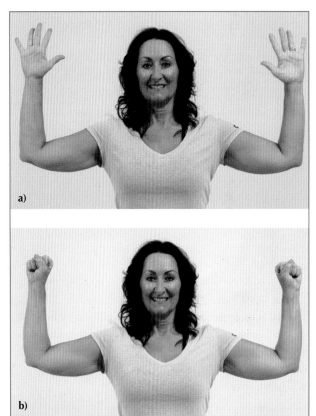

Figure 10.18: *Roos test: (a) Roos position of external rotation at 90 degrees; (b) the patient is asked to open and clench fists for 3 minutes.*

Roos test is performed with the patient seated.

- Instruct the patient to externally rotate and abduct their shoulder to 90 degrees, and also to flex their elbows to 90 degrees (Figure 10.18(a)). This is known as the *I surrender position*.

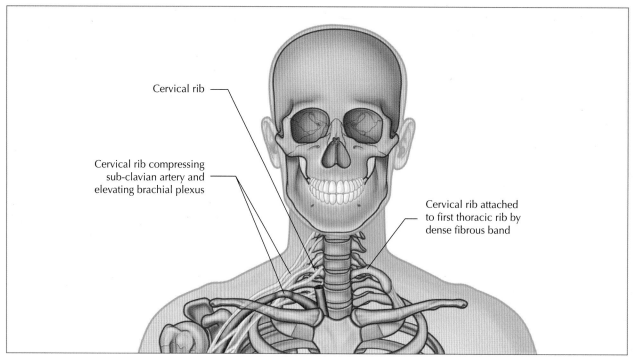

Figure 10.19: *A cervical rib causing TOS.*

- In this position, ask the patient to clench and open their hand at a slow rate (every 2–3 seconds).
- Continue the test for 3 minutes, or until the patient can no longer continue because of pain (Figure 10.18(b)).

According to Gillard et al. (2001), a positive Roos test is the reproduction of pain in the arm, shoulder, chest, or neck; numbness or tingling in the extremity; or an inability to keep up the fist clenching. Roos (1996) suggested that the best positive result is an inability to continue the fist clenching for the full 3 minutes because of pain.

Cervical Ribs and TOS

The natural start of the ribs is at the first thoracic vertebra T1 and the finish is at T12—hence there are 12 pairs of ribs. However, if there is an extra rib present, then this anomaly will be at the level of either the first lumbar vertebra L1 or the seventh cervical vertebra C7; the latter has been suggested as a cause of neurovascular compression at the thoracic outlet (Figure 10.19). The cervical rib can basically be anything from a small stump to a full-size rib that projects from the transverse process of C7, and can even connect to the first thoracic rib by means of a fibrous cartilaginous formation. Some of these extra ribs can be seen on a standard X-ray; unfortunately, some cannot be seen, because not all of these extra ribs calcify and are normally only detected through a surgical procedure.

Scalene Anticus Syndrome and TOS

Howard C. Naffziger (Naffziger and Grant 1938), who was chief of neurosurgery at the University of California, considered the anterior scalene muscle to be the key to the neurovascular compressive abnormalities in patients with cervical rib syndrome, and thus coined the term *scalenus anticus syndrome* (Figure 10.20).

TOS was attributed to spasm and shortening of the anterior scalene muscle, which was believed to develop as a result of a contraction, fibrosis, or hypertrophy of the muscle.

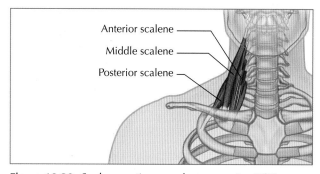

Figure 10.20: *Scalene anticus syndrome causing TOS.*

A former chief of neurological services at the Mayo Clinic called Alfred Adson (Adson and Coffey 1927) began surgically removing the anterior scalene muscle in patients diagnosed with a cervical rib. The compression, he said, originated superiorly and caused the neurovascular structures to press against the bony structure below, and so he felt that the muscle removal operation was safer than resection of the cervical rib.

In reality, the problem is that we inherently use our scalene muscles all the time, so it is easy for them to become short and tight; for instance, if we are a bit anxious, we can end up breathing from our upper chest instead of using our diaphragm. If one has poor posture and has developed a forward head posture with rounded shoulders, the thoracic outlet can become compromised, with trigger points subsequently forming within the shortened scalene muscles.

Costoclavicular Compression Syndrome and TOS

Position wise, the clavicle is parallel to the first rib, and the space formed between these two bony structures is limited. One relatively quick way to test if the clavicle is compressing the underlying rib is through adopting a military or "policeman on parade" type of posture, as shown in Figure 10.21: the shoulders are back and down with the chest out and both arms extended. This exaggerated position stretches as well as compresses the neurovascular bundle (Figure 10.22).

If they wish, the therapist can also palpate the radial pulse at the same time as the patient adopts the military posture. If this military position exacerbates the patient's symptoms by compressing the neurovascular bundle, one can conclude that the clavicle is pressing against the first rib. However, on the odd occasion, the pectoralis minor can also be involved in the compression. If a patient has had a previous clavicle fracture and this has been allowed to heal conservatively rather than being surgically repaired, the additional bone callus that forms might be one reason why the patient is experiencing TOS symptoms.

In 1998, Plewa and Delinger reported that positive test results can be seen as being on a continuum: the loss of radial pulse is the least specific finding (and the most likely to be positive, even in asymptomatic subjects), followed by the production of paresthesia, and then the most specific finding—pain formation in the upper extremity.

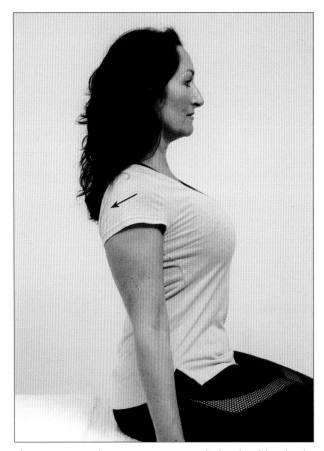

Figure 10.21: *Military-type posture with the shoulders back and down and the chest out.*

Hyperabduction and TOS

The movement of shoulder abduction with end-range flexion (Figure 10.23) can be very relevant to TOS. This particular position might be where the patient needs to place their arm on a daily or regular basis because of their work, and it might well be this continual end-range position that is compromising the neurovascular bundle.

Think about an electrician working on a building site all day every day. He is responsible for placing and wiring all of the ceiling lights in every room, in every house, which means that his arms will be placed above his head for many hours a day on a regular basis. Even though this shoulder position may be the cause of a patient's symptoms, we can use it to our advantage by way of an assessment to decide if the position of hyperabduction exacerbates TOS symptoms.

In this abducted/flexed position the clavicle can approximate the first rib, and the pectoralis minor is considered to be also involved in this position because of

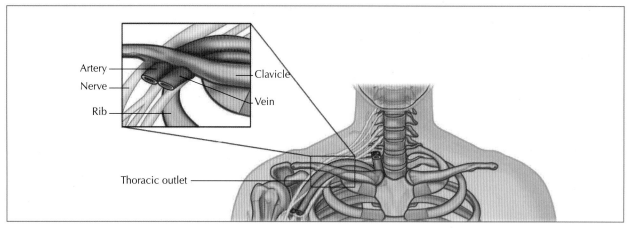

Figure 10.22: *Costoclavicular compression syndrome causing TOS.*

the neurovascular structures passing directly underneath this muscle and the underlying ribs. The position in question causes these structures to be compressed.

Thoracic outlet syndrome (TOS)

Thoracic outlet syndrome (TOS)—PowerPoint

The hyperabduction test is performed with the patient seated.

- Palpate the patient's wrist while you hold their arm in the hyperabduction position (Figure 10.24).
- Ask the patient to let you know if they feel any symptoms, while you also monitor the radial pulse for any changes.
- Hold the position, while the pulse is being monitored, for at least 30 seconds (typically).

When the arms are in an abducted position, the pectoralis minor tendon is stretched and may compress the axillary artery (continuation from the subclavian artery), reducing the strength of the radial pulse and potentially reproducing the presenting symptoms. Malanga et al. (2006) suggest that this test can close down the costoclavicular space, compressing the neurovascular bundle.

Novak et al. (1996) proposed that the test could be enhanced by directing downward pressure to the brachial plexus by digitally pressing just above the clavicle, between the scalene muscles (Figure 10.25).

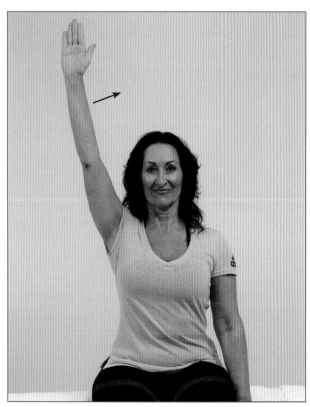

Figure 10.23: *Abduction with end-range flexion compromising the neurovascular bundle.*

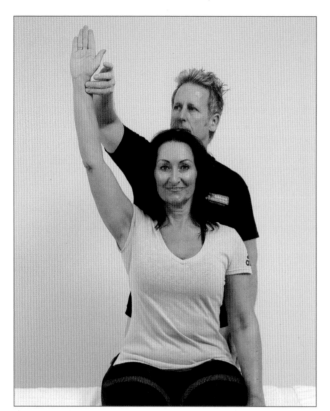

Figure 10.24: *Therapist holds the patient's arm in hyperabduction while palpating the radial pulse.*

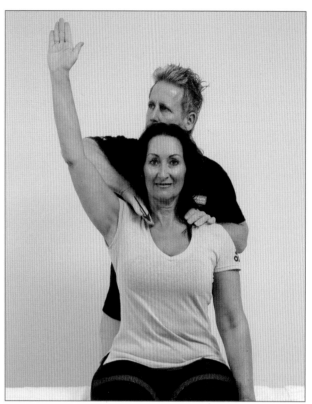

Figure 10.25: *Therapist applies downward pressure to the brachial plexus.*

11

Case Studies of Differential Diagnoses of Musculoskeletal Pain

In this chapter I would like to discuss several individual case studies with you, which I hope you will find of interest. The majority of the patients in question are actually patients who have come to see me personally at my clinic at the University of Oxford. The reason for discussing these cases is that I have been lecturing in the fields of sports medicine and manual therapy for many years now, and during this time I have come to realize that many practitioners in physical therapy sadly treat the area where the patient presents with pain, rather than considering if this is the actual cause of the patient's problem or if it is merely a symptom. The potential for the referral of pain from systemic disease via the neurological system to specific muscles and joints is well documented in the medical literature. These referral patterns most often affect the back and shoulder, but may also appear in the chest, thorax, hip, groin, or even sacroiliac joint.

It is essential that all therapists take a thorough case history of each and every patient, and then correlate their subjective and objective findings in order to recognize presenting conditions that might require medical referral. The therapist should conduct a systems review (heart and lungs, gastrointestinal screening, etc.), and needs to be familiar with different types of pain, specific pain patterns, and any types of sign and symptom that may suggest systemic origins of problems that could potentially appear within the musculoskeletal system.

When I teach any of the master class courses at my clinic at the University of Oxford, the audience is generally students from all corners of the earth—a fact that makes me feel truly honored. During these classes, I regularly discuss differential diagnosis of musculoskeletal pain, and I have often found it disappointing how little knowledge many physical therapists have regarding other bodily structures and vital organs (viscera or viscus) that can be the underlying causative factor in the patient's presenting symptoms (or at least contribute to them).

Medically trained personnel, whose initial training is generally longer, may have greater knowledge but hopefully this chapter will appeal to all readers and serve as a reminder of the specific conditions, especially from and via the neurological system, that can cause pain as well as other types of symptom to other areas of the body. It is very important that a symptom of pain with a musculoskeletal origin be differentiated from pain arising from a visceral condition. Why? Because the two types of pain can readily mimic each other in terms of how they present, as we will read shortly.

My personal belief about any form of assessment of the musculoskeletal system tends to chime with a methodology that was taught to me many years ago when I was student of osteopathy—namely, the *KISS principle* (I mentioned this earlier, in Chapter 9). In other words, try not to complicate matters too much when discussing the patient's presenting symptoms. If we ask the right type of question, hopefully we will receive the right type of answer. The same principle applies to the subjective assessment—if possible, try to methodically run through the appropriate testing procedures, rather than utilizing all the tests under the sun.

Case Studies 11.1–11.11, as I said earlier, mainly relate to actual patients who attended my clinic at Oxford.

The reader is encouraged to contemplate some of the *key factors* for these patients; there are clues as to what is going on in both the subjective history and medical history. Consider what you feel is the likely cause of the patient's pain before going on to review some of the hypotheses proposed according to my own personal beliefs pertaining to each of the complaints.

■ Swallowing Food Causes Unusual Reaction

CASE STUDY 11.1

A student who I taught a few years ago and lives locally to me in Oxfordshire asked me to have a look at one of his patients, as nobody had been able to help him. The presenting condition was unique to me, as I have never encountered it before. Basically, whenever the patient swallowed food, he would experience pain in his left forearm! This had been ongoing for over two years, and every single time this gentleman swallowed, regardless of the type of food, the pain in his arm would manifest. He had seen numerous members of the medical profession, but they were all basically confused and could not give him a reason why this was happening to him. He even had camera investigations of his throat, esophagus, and stomach by two different surgeons, but nothing was found to be wrong, and the cause of his symptoms could not be explained. Both the surgeons believed surgery might be helpful, although they were not exactly sure about which structure/s to operate on, and naturally there was a high risk that surgery would not change his symptoms.

When he initially emailed me, one of the first things that went through my mind, especially as I call myself a "therapy detective," was that the problem might be coming from the cervical spine; I thought the pain he perceived to be referring to the dermatome of his forearm. If that was the case, was the issue possibly originating from the nerve root level C6 or even C7? The patient in question said he had had an MRI scan a few weeks ago and that there was nothing of real concern; however, the scan did show a disc bulge at the level C6/7 that was protruding into the left intervertebral foramen, with light contact to the left exiting nerve root of C7.

I won't lie to you about this condition, as I had personally never encountered it before—the symptoms were new to me but I did find it intriguing. Maybe, just maybe,

there was a connection with swallowing, and somehow that motion was exacerbating the disc bulge that was subsequently referring to the C7 dermatome of his forearm.

In terms of the assessment, the reflexes for C5/6/7 on the left and right sides of his upper limb tested normal (2++), and even the myotome for all the areas of C5–T1 tested strong (Grade 5). That, in itself, was a little confusing and almost disappointing, as I wanted to find something that was obviously wrong! However, upon applying palpation techniques, I did feel a restriction in the left side of the lower part of his cervical spine, around C6/7; I proceeded to perform a spinal manipulative technique to the area of C6/7, whereby an audible cavitation was heard.

The patient messaged me a few days later saying that they felt their symptoms had subsided a little, but were still very much there. I have seen this patient a few times since, and I am pleased to say that they have improved overall since the initial consultation.

Case Study 11.1, in particular, was very memorable, and will stay with me for many years to come, especially as I have encountered, and had discussions with, over one hundred thousand particular cases. I like to think that every patient has their own unique story to tell, and I personally believe that in Case Study 11.1, I was at least able to assist and reduce some of the patient's presenting symptoms through my treatment protocols. This patient is still coming to the clinic for treatment, because his symptoms are still present when he swallows food. But, fingers crossed, with ongoing treatment he will improve to the point that he will be discharged from the clinic.

■ Arm Abduction Induces Shoulder Shrugging

CASE STUDY 11.2

The patient here is a 45-year-old male who presented to the clinic and said to me that he could not lift his arm (abduct) to the side without shrugging his shoulder to compensate. Every morning after waking up, the first thing this patient would do was lie down and adopt a prone position on the floor, and perform 50 push-ups. However, about three weeks prior to his appointment with me, he was doing the push-ups as normal but suddenly felt pain in his shoulder on just the fourth repetition, and had to stop because his arm was so painful.

When I assessed him and specifically asked him to show me what he could not do, he tried to abduct, or even simply flex, his shoulder. I noticed that there was no active contraction of the deltoid muscle, and observed that the other muscles, such as the supraspinatus and pectoralis major, were overly compensating. Perhaps this was the reason why he could not lift his arm—because his deltoid was unable to contract. The patient also had some strange feelings just above where the deltoid inserts (the "regimental badge" area). Let me give you an example of this altered sensation: if I touched this area lightly (say with a piece of cotton wool or with my finger tip), the patient would back off and say it hurts, even though I was touching him extremely lightly.

My hypothesis for this patient was that something (presumably the push-up) had caused an increased motion of the humeral head, which had subsequently damaged his axillary nerve. This nerve supplies the deltoid as well as the teres minor, which would explain why he had the strange symptoms in the "regimental badge" area (think back to Chapter 10)—this specific area is related to the axillary nerve. In terms of treatment, I advised him that, with some mobilizations and soft-tissue work, the nerve would hopefully regenerate, although this healing mechanism might take a few months (recall, nerve regeneration is approximately 0.04″ (1mm) per day, or 1″ (2.5cm) per month). I am pleased to say that this was indeed the case, as four months later, the patient regained full motion and power.

Regarding Case Study 11.2, many therapists with a good knowledge base might say it could be a C5 (cervical level 5, between the C4/5 region) nerve root problem that is potentially causing weakness in shoulder abduction, which is a perfectly valid theory. However, the C5 myotome also innervates the motion of elbow flexion, but here the patient tested strong for contraction of the biceps muscle. Furthermore, there was no weakness in other C5-innervated muscles, such as the supraspinatus or infraspinatus. In this case, therefore, it cannot be a C5 nerve root issue.

I used to be a vehicle electrician when I was in the military, and I think of the axillary nerve as a sidelight or indicator on an automobile: if the bulb has blown or the electric wire has been cut (open circuit), the light will

cease to function. In the case of the axillary nerve, if the nerve (the electric wire) that supplies the deltoid and teres minor muscles has been damaged, this can subsequently cause the nerve to switch off and the muscles to become inhibited (the light bulb goes off or dims). As a result, the muscles in question will test weak and start to atrophy (waste away) very quickly. However, everything else in the body (the car) will work as normal, and initially you might not notice a problem. It will not be long, though, before you become aware of the issue.

■ Armpit Pain Restricts Gym Workouts

CASE STUDY 11.3

A 49-year-old male presented with pain in his left axilla (armpit area), which radiated into his left anterior chest. The onset was six weeks ago, with no obvious cause. The pain was worse at night, and the patient found it difficult to adopt a position that eased the pain. He had reduced his gym activity because he considered that exercising was exacerbating the pain he perceived in the axillary region. AROM of his shoulder joint and cervical spine caused no pain or revealed any signs of being restricted.

Medical History

The patient has had a cardiac examination, including an electrocardiogram (ECG), and this was all clear. There is a history of a hiatus hernia about a year ago, for which he is on medication.

Hypothesis:

- Rotator cuff strain?
- Cervical referred pain?
- Serratus anterior strain?
- Frozen shoulder (adhesive capsulitis)?
- Lung, rib, intercostals issue?
- Lymphatic node enlargement?

Before I discuss my own hypothesis, it is first necessary to support or reject the hypotheses listed above. Taking into consideration the patient's history, it is worth noting that his shoulder and cervical spine have no particular restrictions and do not refer pain or exacerbate any of his symptoms. There is no history of trauma or overuse, so muscular causes can be ruled out. Inhalation, coughing, or sneezing has no effect on his pain, so again this rules out the intervertebral discs, lungs, ribs, etc. There is no apparent swelling in his axilla and there are no infections, so we can safely rule out inflamed lymph nodes.

The obvious give away to me can be found in his case history: he experiences pain at night and, more importantly, cannot find a position that eases his symptoms. This is generally what would be known as a *red flag* and requires further investigation, as it can indicate some form of carcinoma (cancer). This patient, however, had no other symptoms and was otherwise perfectly healthy, so I did not consider a referral was necessary at this stage.

My hypothesis for the diagnosis was that the *hiatus hernia* was the cause of his night pain, as this was referring into his mid-thoracic spine via the sympathetic nervous system (think back to Chapter 2 on the peripheral nervous system). It was causing the vertebral segment to become *facilitated,* which I then considered was being referred to his axilla by the thoracic vertebra; this is known as a *visceral-somatic dysfunction* (*viscera* = "organs"; *soma* = "body"). The patient responded successfully to osteopathic treatment that focused mainly on his thoracic spine, as well as modifications to his daily diet.

■ Pain on Top of Shoulder Disrupts Sleep

CASE STUDY 11.4

A lady in her mid-40s presented to the clinic with pain generally located on the top of her right shoulder, and in particular in the region of her upper trapezius muscle. This had been present for many months with no obvious cause. During the day, the lady was not aware of her pain, but at night, while she was sleeping, the right shoulder became noticeably worse, to the point that she would wake up, take some medication, and eventually fall back to sleep. She also mentioned that something was not quite right with her middle to lower thoracic spine, but said that her shoulder pain was the priority.

On examination, I asked the lady to abduct her shoulder as far as it felt comfortable, and to my surprise, she could easily reach a full ROM of 180 degrees. It was the same when she was asked to flex her shoulder: she also managed to reach the full 180 degrees of motion with no issues. I then asked her to circle her arm forward and backward a few times, and she surprised me again by performing

these movements pain free and with no symptoms. Because the lady could abduct and flex her shoulder through full range, I considered that there could not be any underlying musculoskeletal issue present that was directly related to the region of the shoulder complex.

This next sentence or two might sound a bit strange, as I asked the patient the following: "When you go to the toilet, have you noticed that your stool has a tendency to float on the surface, rather than sinking to the bottom of the bowl?" As expected, the lady looked a little startled, but responded: "Funny you should ask that question—yes, my stool does seem to float when I go to the toilet."

Before I continue with the case study, ask yourself why I enquired about this delicate subject—what do you think was going through my mind? Before I answer this question, I would like to mention something that was taught to me when I was studying osteopathy. One particular lecture that I found extremely fascinating, and remembered vividly because I was so interested in the topic, was about differential diagnosis of musculoskeletal pain in physical therapy. The lecturer had talked about a female patient who presented to him with right-sided shoulder pain *and* who surprisingly had full ROM without any pain in all the tested movements. The lecturer proceeded to discuss something known as the *four Fs*—female, fair, fat, and forty. You can probably guess that this decidedly outdated turn of phrase relates to an overweight lady with fair hair who is approaching middle age. My patient certainly fitted this profile.

To cut a long story short, the tutor was saying that if a patient comes to your clinic with right-sided shoulder pain and fits the criteria of the four Fs, then you need to consider that the gallbladder might be the underlying causative factor for the patient's presenting symptoms of pain in the right shoulder. Common conditions that occur with the gallbladder are inflammation (cholecystitis) and gallstones (cholelithiasis).

I am anticipating at this point that I have whet your appetite enough for you to want to gain more underpinning knowledge of the subject in question here. Hopefully, you are now trying to work out in your head the answer to the following question: "How does the gallbladder organ cause right-sided shoulder pain?"

The link is the proximity of a nerve called the *phrenic nerve* and its relationship to the gallbladder. The phrenic nerve innervates the central component of the respiratory muscle, the diaphragm (it is a musculotendinous structure and not a viscus). This nerve originates from the cervical levels C3, C4, and C5, and there is a simple mnemonic to remember this: "C3, 4, 5, keep the diaphragm alive" (see Chapter 3). This relates to spinal cord trauma, in that if you damage the spinal cord below the level of C5, you should be able to breathe on your own unassisted; however, if you damage the spinal cord above the level of C3, you might need to have artificial respiration. The peripheral part of the diaphragm, on the other hand, is innervated by the lower six intercostal nerves, and consequently does not refer pain to the shoulder complex.

Gallbladder Inflammation

Let us now look at the scenario of an inflamed gallbladder. Because of the gallbladder's close proximity to the diaphragm and the phrenic nerve (Figure 11.1(a)), there is a stimulus that excites the neurological system, and a signal is subsequently relayed back to the origins of the nerve located in the C3–5 cervical spine region. If you look at the innervation of the diaphragm and the map of the neurological dermatomes, you will notice that C3–5 actually covers the area of the upper limb, and, in particular, the shoulder region (Figure 11.1(b)).

Note: The supraclavicular nerve (C3, 4) is responsible for the pain referred to in shoulder tip pain, and it is the peritoneum, supplied by the phrenic nerve, that is stimulated. It is *not* the organ giving pain, but the irritation of the overlying peritoneum supplied by somatic nerves.

Pain that is referred from the diaphragm is typically felt near the superior angle of the scapula, along the suprascapular

fossa, and even along the upper trapezius muscle; it can be exacerbated when the patient coughs, sneezes, or takes deep breaths. What I am saying is the following. If you have a pathological issue with your gallbladder, the chances of having right shoulder pain are increased, because the pain signals are transmitted back to the cervical spine, and the sensory input is then transported to the peripheral nerve and subsequently to the dermatomes.

One could view this as a *referred pattern of pain*. Let me give you an example: someone is having a myocardial infarction (heart attack). This person will naturally feel intense pain in the central chest region, but in general patients describe feeling pain or sensations in other areas too—mid-thoracic spine, left arm and hand, and even on the left side of the face and jaw.

What I would like to do now is suggest an analogy for the heart attack process. Imagine you are traveling to London by train on a Monday morning at rush hour, arriving at, say, Paddington station. Hundreds of people will all get off the carriages at the same time. The conductor will direct them through the normal gates (relate the flow of people to chest pain). Nevertheless, because so many people are getting off the train, a queue forms, and now the conductor diverts some people to alternative gates (left side of the face and jaw). If these gates too become busy, people are redirected to yet another gate (arm and hand), which might be a few extra minutes' walk away. I hope that this analogy makes some sense to you.

Simply put, if the gallbladder becomes inflamed, pain can be referred to the right shoulder via the phrenic nerve, as well as to the area of the mid- to lower thoracic spine.

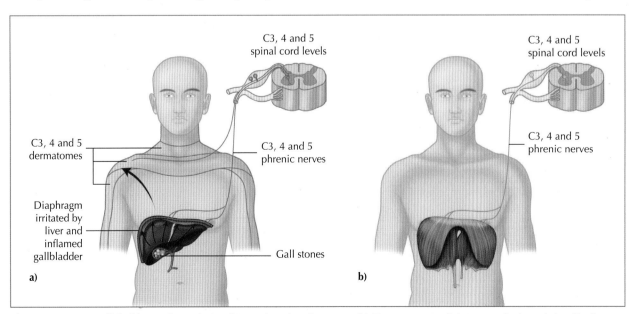

Figure 11.1: *(a) Gallbladder and its relationship to the phrenic nerve. (b) Dermatomes of the upper limb and the diaphragm.*

This occurs because of the sympathetic nerve celiac ganglia innervation of the gallbladder. Furthermore, because of the proximity of the gallbladder to the abdomen, the patient could perceive pain in the right lower costal margin, which is located in the right upper quadrant of the abdomen.

There is a small area under the right lower costal margin (rib) that, when palpated (especially with the patient breathing in), may cause a rebound tenderness (Figure 11.2). This is known as *Murphy's sign* and is a positive finding for an inflamed gallbladder, especially if the same procedure is performed on the left side of the abdomen with no pain perceived by the patient.

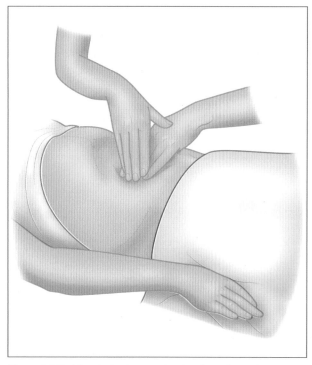

Figure 11.2: *Murphy's sign—palpation for rebound tenderness, indicating a gallbladder condition.*

Conclusion

Regarding the lady in Case Study 11.4, I mentioned to her that I thought the gallbladder was responsible for the pain in her right shoulder, as well as for the discomfort in her mid- to lower thoracic spine. I discussed with her the function of the gallbladder in terms of breaking down fatty foods, etc., and said that if this organ does not function correctly, stool has a tendency to float. I also explained, through anatomical books and diagrams, how the gallbladder caused the pain in her right shoulder via the phrenic nerve.

I wrote a letter to the patient's doctor, setting forth my findings, and the patient was referred to a gastrointestinal consultant, who confirmed it was a gallbladder condition and removed the organ in due course. The patient in question had a follow-up appointment with me a few weeks after the surgery, and I was pleased to see that her shoulder and thoracic pain had disappeared.

This type of condition is what is described as a *visceral-somatic dysfunction* because the viscus (organ) is the underlying causative factor for pain to present itself to the somatic/soma region (body)—in this case the right shoulder.

With regard to a gallbladder condition, patients can also present with right upper abdominal pain, as well as nausea and vomiting, after eating fatty meals. They might also present with jaundice, low-grade fever, and weight loss, especially if some form of cancer is present.

Liver Association with Gallbladder

The liver can suffer from conditions such as cirrhosis, tumors, and hepatitis (*hepatic* = relating to the liver), and this organ has an association with the gallbladder and the common bile duct (biliary = relating to bile). These organs commonly present with musculoskeletal symptoms in the right shoulder and upper trapezius regions, because of the liver's contact with the central portion of the diaphragm, thoracic spine, and interscapular regions of the upper body (Figure 11.3), as well as with pain in the right upper quadrant of the abdomen. The liver is the most common site for secondary cancer metastasis (especially in men older than 50) as a result of other primary cancer sites, such as the stomach, lung, and pancreas, and the breast in women.

The sympathetic nerve fibers from the hepatic and biliary systems are connected through the splanchnic and celiac plexuses, and have their origins in the thoracic spine, potentially producing interscapular pain and possibly intercostal pain. The splanchnic nerves synapse with the phrenic nerve, hence producing pain in the region of the right shoulder.

From a practitioner perspective, the physical therapist might be the first person to see this patient presenting with what they think is a simple musculoskeletal problem in the right shoulder. It is of paramount importance that a detailed case history be taken, making close observations of the patient's physical appearance and well-being, and looking for any obvious skin changes. The physical therapist will need to diversify and ask appropriate non-musculoskeletal questions that relate to the urinary

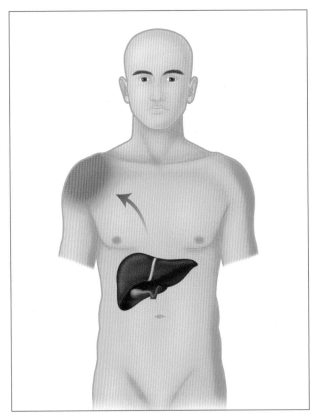

Figure 11.3: *Pain sites originating from the liver, gallbladder, and common bile duct.*

and gastrointestinal systems. For example, one of the functions of the liver, or biliary system, is to combine bile with bilirubin, which gives the stool its natural brown color. If, as a result of some pathology, these systems lose the ability to excrete bilirubin, then the color of the urine can change and become dark, almost like the color of cola or tea. This also has the effect of changing the stool from its normal brown appearance to a light color.

■ Referred Pain to Shoulder After Rugby Tackle

CASE STUDY 11.5

The person in this case study did not visit the clinic to see me, rather I was actually training someone on a shoulder course and they mentioned it to the class. I thought it was so interesting that I should include it, as I am sure it will help you understand other causes of referred pain.

The patient in question was a young male who, while playing rugby one Sunday afternoon, was tackled and hit the ground hard, landing on the left side of his body and feeling pretty winded. The physiotherapist providing

medical cover for the match gave him some assistance and said it would be best if he came off the pitch to rest a while. After the game, the player complained of left shoulder pain, and the therapist thought he might have damaged his rotator cuff and prescribed him some strengthening exercises.

Despite having a restful night, the player woke up the next day with severe pain in his left shoulder but still managed to go to work. While he was sitting at his desk, he collapsed and was rushed to the hospital emergency department, where he was diagnosed with a ruptured spleen.

Think back to the proximity of the phrenic nerve to the various organs explained earlier. Relevant to this particular case, the spleen is located on the left side of the body, at a similar level to that of the gallbladder and the liver on the right side. A damaged or ruptured spleen can also refer pain, but this time to the left shoulder (Figure 11.4) rather than the right, as in the earlier Case Study 11.4. However, the C3–5 dermatomes are still involved because of the relationship to the phrenic nerve, with the subsequent referral pattern to the region of the left shoulder.

There are a multitude of problems that present to therapists, especially in a sporting context, and it is very

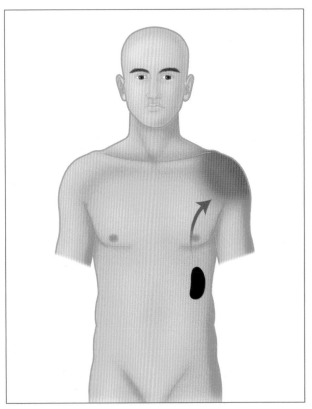

Figure 11.4: *Pain sites referred from the spleen.*

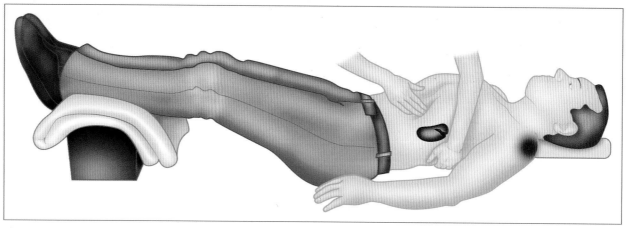

Figure 11.5: *Kehr's sign and the relationship to the spleen.*

easy to come to a diagnosis of a rotator cuff tear when a player complains of shoulder pain. However, if the physiotherapist had assessed the player fully, they would have probably seen a full ROM in abduction and flexion of the shoulder complex, without any pain. That in itself should have been a red flag for a medical referral.

Moreover, this particular patient had a history of trauma with a sudden onset of symptoms, especially with left shoulder pain. Knowledge of the patient's history in this case would therefore have been beneficial and might have suggested an initial referral for at least a second opinion. A sign called *Kehr's sign* relates to pain that typically presents itself at the tip of the shoulder (Figure 11.5), and the most common cause of this pain in the left shoulder is a ruptured spleen.

■ Chronic Shoulder Pain and Loss of Dexterity

CASE STUDY 11.6

A 68-year-old woman was referred by her local doctor to a physiotherapy clinic for treatment of chronic shoulder pain. She had a 12-week ongoing history of constant severe pain in her right shoulder; this pain also radiated beneath her scapula, into her right axilla, and around the right side of her chest wall. She mentioned an awareness of shortness of breath and complained of increased pain and chest tightness, especially when deep breathing. Walking a short distance, sitting, and even turning over in bed exacerbated the pain. On further questioning, she also reported that she had a reduced appetite, as well as sleep disturbance due to the discomfort, and that she was a long-term heavy smoker.

On examination, this patient was found to have a "normal" shoulder in terms of ROM, but there were some cervical and thoracic spine movements that were restricted and painful; this was considered to be caused by age-related degenerative changes. There was no arm pain or paresthesia; however, the patient mentioned that her right hand had symptoms of grip weakness, loss of dexterity, and a feeling of her arm "not belonging to her." However, on neurological testing there was no deficit in reflex testing, nor was there any obvious weakness of the muscles in the upper limbs associated with the corresponding myotomes for C5–7.

The patient had private health insurance and requested an MRI scan rather than a standard X-ray as soon as possible, because she was naturally worried about her symptoms. The medical diagnosis was a large Pancoast tumor (it was probably the compression from this tumor in the lower brachial plexus of C8/T1—ulnar nerve—that was causing the loss of dexterity). Unfortunately, because of the size of the tumor, it was considered inoperable, so palliative care was given; the lady passed away a few months later. The patient did not present with Horner's syndrome in this instance, because the tumor had not progressed far enough to compress the paravertebral sympathetic nerves.

■ Painful Right Shoulder and Coughing

CASE STUDY 11.7

A 42-year-old neighbor was referred to me by his wife, as she was annoyed that he kept complaining about his painful right shoulder, especially in his trapezius area, but would do nothing about it. This had been going on for a few months, and she suspected that it might be a neck problem, because he had some history of neck pain from time to time. As I lived close by, she thought it would make sense to come to see me. However, I was out of the country lecturing at the time and said I would see him on my return.

A week or so later, his wife emailed me, saying her husband now had a painful persistent cough and what did I think. I immediately replied that he needed to see his doctor at once for further investigation, because I considered a lung X-ray essential in order to rule out any sinister condition, especially with his new symptoms and him being an ex-smoker.

Unfortunately, my hypothesis was correct, as the patient was diagnosed with a stage 3 Pancoast tumor. Since the diagnosis, he has undergone chemotherapy and radiotherapy, and after many months passed, he was fortunately given the all clear. However, the life of this patient has completely changed (maybe for the better in one respect): he no longer takes anything for granted, because he has realized that life is so short and can be taken away at any moment.

Just think about Case Study 11.7 for a second, and I say this to all my students: on the face of it, this case appears to be straightforward in terms of assessment and subsequent treatment of the area of the upper trapezius muscle as well as his neck for what he initially presented with. I too would have been no different in my approach and would have treated the same muscles, had I not known that there was anything sinister present that was responsible for his musculoskeletal pain presentation. However, things suddenly changed for me as soon as he mentioned a persistent and painful cough, as this was definitely a red flag condition, signaling that a medical referral was essential.

Lung Carcinoma (Pancoast Tumor)

A US radiologist called Henry Pancoast described a type of lung cancer termed a *Pancoast tumor*, which is defined primarily by its location at the extreme apex (very top) of the right or left lung (Figure 11.6). The reason I am writing about lung carcinoma and the shoulder is because of the relationship to the lower roots of the brachial plexus and subclavian artery. As the Pancoast tumor progresses, the nerves and blood vessels can be affected, potentially mimicking a thoracic outlet syndrome (TOS). Thus, the patient can present with pain in the areas of the shoulder, axilla, scapula, arm, and hand, as well as with atrophy/weakness of the hand and arm muscles. Because of the location of this type of tumor within the apex, it is less likely to cause the typical symptoms seen with lung cancer, such as shortness of breath, persistent cough, and coughing up blood.

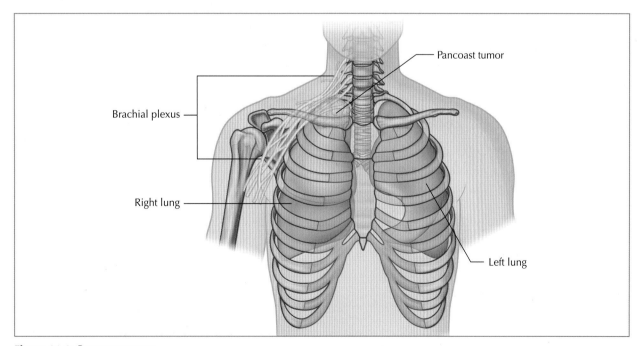

Figure 11.6: *Pancoast tumor.*

Typically, the later stages of a Pancoast tumor cause *Horner's syndrome* (Figure 11.7), because of compression of the sympathetic ganglion. The symptoms of a Pancoast tumor in severe cases include drooping of the eyelid (ptosis), constriction of the pupil (miosis), and lack of sweating on one side of the face (anhidrosis). Other symptoms are unexplained weight loss, loss of appetite, fatigue, sleep disturbance, chest tightness, and arm or hand weakness and a flushed face due to lack of vasoconstriction.

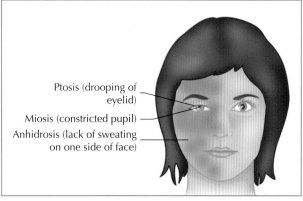

Ptosis (drooping of eyelid)

Miosis (constricted pupil)

Anhidrosis (lack of sweating on one side of face)

Figure 11.7: *Horner's syndrome.*

■ Increased Upper Back Pain After a Beer and Curry

CASE STUDY 11.8

A man in his mid-twenties came to my clinic presenting with pain in his mid- to lower thoracic spine; he also mentioned being aware that something that was not quite right in his right shoulder, but he could not say quite what exactly. These symptoms had been present for many months and did not give the impression of going away anytime soon.

During the medical screening, I asked him about specific things that exacerbated his symptoms, and he replied, smiling, saying that "beer and curries" seemed to make his symptoms feel worse. I asked him how often he partook of these, and he said that he had a few beers every evening and frequently enjoyed a spicy curry.

When I assessed the patient and focused initially on the area of his thoracic spine, I found that he had particular spinal restrictions and tenderness in the area of T4–9. I also noticed that the skin overlying that area of the spine had trophic changes (dry, scaly, pimply skin) and became hyperemic

(an excess of blood, causing reddening of the skin) quite quickly on light palpation. The muscles overlying the thoracic spine felt very firm to the touch, and I considered them to be hypertonic (in an increased state of contraction).

I told this gentleman to see his general practitioner, because I felt that there could be the possibility of him having an *ulcer* and that this was responsible for his presenting symptoms (Figure 11.8). I also said that physical therapy in this instance would probably not be of any value. The patient telephoned me a few weeks later and confirmed my diagnosis of an ulcer, the cause being an infection due to a type of bacteria called *Helicobacter pylori (H. pylori)*. He was put on medication for the infection, and I am pleased to say that he has also reduced his regular intake of alcohol and curries. I am hoping that in time he will make a full recovery.

Regarding Case Study 11.8, the trophic changes to the patient's thoracic spine were related to the sympathetic nerves from the stomach and small intestine being overstimulated, a condition called *sympathetictonia*

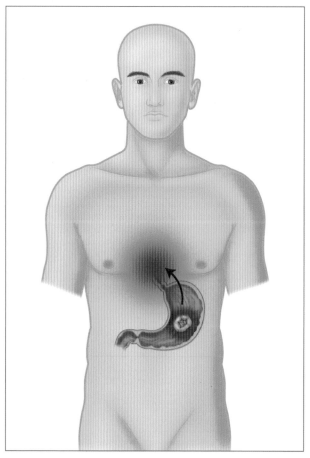

Figure 11.8: *Stomach ulcer and thoracic pain.*

(increased tone of the sympathetic nervous system). This condition alters the tone of the overlying muscles, as well as affecting the function of the sebaceous glands and hair follicles. In my medical notes, I remember writing down he presented with a visceral-somatic dysfunction that was responsible for causing pain in the soma (body), and the underlying cause was more than likely to be a peptic ulcer.

Both the stomach and small intestine (duodenum) can be a source of pain in the right shoulder, particularly in the superior angle of the scapula as well as the suprascapular region and the upper trapezius muscle. A *H. pylori* infection is commonly considered to be the main cause of the majority of abdominal conditions that are specifically related to gastric or duodenal ulcers. Approximately 10% of ulcers result from the chronic use of nonsteroidal anti-inflammatory drugs (NSAIDs), such as ibuprofen, naproxen, and aspirin, which are often taken long term for arthritic types of medical condition.

The physical therapist has to be continually aware of other presenting signs and symptoms, because pain located in the midline of the epigastrium or upper abdomen, as well as pain in the right shoulder, could possibly be referred from the gallbladder and liver as well as from the stomach or small intestine. An intuitive approach through correct questioning during the initial history taking is essential, because there are almost certainly other signs and symptoms present that are associated with the above-mentioned organs. For example: "Does the pain change during specific times, such as when eating meals?" or "Have you noticed your stool is particularly dark?" (this darkness within the stool is called a *melena*, and can relate to bleeding in the upper section of the alimentary canal, stomach, or small intestine).

■ Swelling Above Left Clavicle

CASE STUDY 11.9

I have had the privilege of knowing a very good friend for over ten years, and I will call him Mark (renamed here to hide his true identity). Mark was a physical therapist who lived in Wales, and when he approached his sixties, he decided to do an online test for colon cancer; unfortunately, he tested positive for a carcinoma. Over the next few months he had the majority of his colon removed, with continual chemotherapy and radiotherapy treatments. I saw Mark a year or so after his diagnosis and he was a changed man: he must have lost over four stone (26kg) in weight. The months passed and everything seemed to be going well.

When Mark attended a course with me in Oxford in November that year, he mentioned a swelling above his left clavicle (supraclavicular fossa) and complained of left shoulder and arm discomfort. The doctor had put him on medication, and he could not venture into the sunlight because of the prescribed medication. The doctors had found something in his left lung, but did not actually say what they had found, only that further tests were necessary.

I thought to myself that this would probably be the last time I would see my good friend, and not surprisingly, this was true: in late December he passed away. The diagnosis was actually a stomach carcinoma, which was most likely related to the initial primary colon cancer causing secondary cancers that had metastasized to his stomach and lung. The swelling that was present in his left supraclavicular fossa was probably due to metastasizing enlargements of the lymph nodes from the stomach cancer.

Virchow's Node

It is a known fact that a swelling in the left supraclavicular fossa can be one of the first signs of stomach cancer, and that malignancies of the stomach can actually be asymptomatic and reach an advanced stage before producing any symptoms. The particular left-side lymph node involved is called *Virchow's node* (named in 1848 after the German pathologist Rudolf Virchow), and has the scary alternative name of the *devil's lymph node*, for obvious reasons.

The thoracic duct (left side), shown in Figure 11.9, in relation to the lymphatic system is like a reservoir (unlike the right side); it is responsible for draining the lymphatic fluid for the majority of the body before it enters the subclavian veins of the venous system. If there are metastases present, the thoracic duct can become blocked, which causes a regurgitation of the lymphatic fluid into the Virchow's lymph node (Figure 11.9).

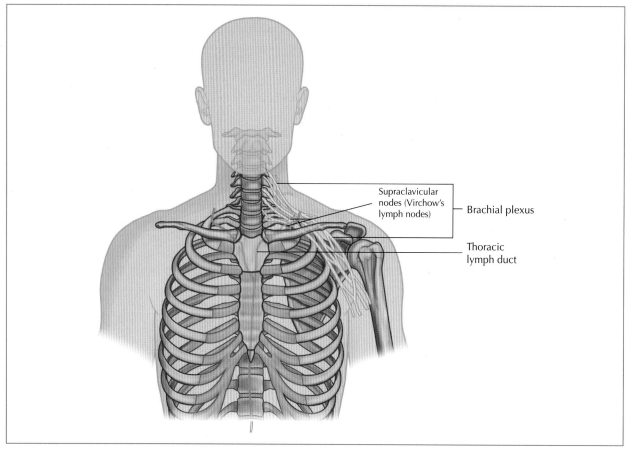

Supraclavicular nodes (Virchow's lymph nodes)

Brachial plexus

Thoracic lymph duct

Figure 11.9: *Thoracic lymph duct and Virchow's lymph node.*

■ Left Shoulder, Abdominal, and Back Pain

CASE STUDY 11.10

One of the therapists whom I had had the privilege of teaching emailed me, saying that she had a patient who presented with left shoulder pain as well as abdominal and back pain; the patient also reported increased weight loss over a short period of time. The doctor had told the patient it was indigestion and sent her home.

The therapist was concerned it was more than just indigestion, however, and sent her back to the doctor the next day. After further investigations, the patient was diagnosed with pancreatic cancer and unfortunately passed away not long after she was given the full diagnosis.

The therapist in question messaged me the following week to say that she had another patient with similar symptoms. This patient, a male in his fifties who played badminton four times a week and cycled a lot, came to her clinic presenting with symptoms mainly in his left groin, which were relieved by him "curling up." He also mentioned left shoulder and some abdominal symptoms. He too was referred to the doctor and was unfortunately diagnosed with pancreatic cancer, sadly passing away a few weeks later.

Pancreas

Generally speaking, the pancreas, especially in the case of a pancreatic carcinoma rather than pancreatitis (inflammation), can be nonspecific and rather vague in terms of the presenting signs and symptoms (Figure 11.10). It has been clinically proven that lower back pain may be the only symptom that patients present with. I can guarantee that if a patient walks into the clinic and presents with lower back pain, the majority of physical therapists and medical practitioners will *not* suspect pancreatic carcinoma, and will consider other musculoskeletal causes of their back pain. However, the presence of the following signs and symptoms should arouse suspicion:

- Upper abdominal pain (epigastric) that radiates into the back
- Unexplained weight loss and loss of appetite
- Light-colored stools
- Dark urine
- Constipation
- Nausea and vomiting
- Lower back pain
- Left shoulder pain
- Jaundice

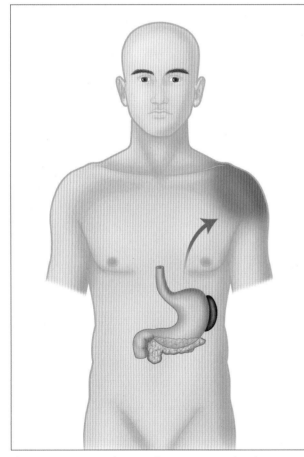

Figure 11.10: *Typical areas of pain associated with the pancreas.*

Patients with a condition of their pancreas tend to find relief by bending forward and bringing their knees to their chest (curling up), while symptoms are sometimes exacerbated by drinking alcohol, eating food, and even walking or lying flat (supine) with the legs straight.

Over the last few years, I have lectured to many thousands of therapists from all corners of the earth. In these courses I have rarely spoken about the pancreas causing shoulder, back, and groin pain via the neurological system. This is mainly because I have so much information to cover in one day that it is difficult to include every single thing that therapists might see in their practice—the course would end up taking five days rather than one. From now on, however, I can promise you that, when teaching my master classes, I will always talk about the pancreas. It gives me no end of satisfaction when I look back at the email I received from my previous student and see that she remembered me mentioning the shoulder pain/cancer link during the workshop she had taken. I am very pleased to say that at least some of the knowledge I pass on can be of value.

Kidney

I have personally seen thousands of patients, and I cannot recall any one of these having upper limb pain that was directly related to a kidney condition. Then again, perhaps in my earlier years of training, I might have missed this underlying causative factor of symptoms in the shoulder.

The kidney will potentially only cause ipsilateral (same side) shoulder pain if it contacts and causes increased pressure to the diaphragm (even though this is a rare symptom for any type of kidney condition), and we know about the relationship to the phrenic nerve (discussed previously—see chapters 3 and 10 and Case Study 11.4).

It is not within the scope of this text to go through all the specific medical conditions that relate to the renal and urologic systems; however, some of the signs and symptoms might be of concern to the physical therapist. Renal pain is commonly felt in the posterior subcostal and costovertebral regions (Figure 11.11). The pain can also be felt around the flank, into the lower abdominal quadrant, and even radiating into the testicular/genitalia area. As you can see from Figure 11.11, lower back pain and possibly ipsilateral shoulder pain may also be present.

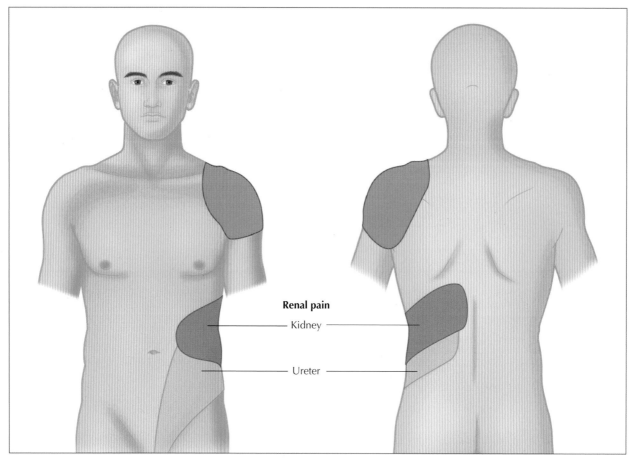

Renal pain

— Kidney —

— Ureter —

Figure 11.11: *Typical areas associated with renal and urologic pain.*

■ Sciatica-type Pain After Short Walks

CASE STUDY 11.11

Many years ago, a 60-year-old slim-looking male came to the clinic presenting with generalized sciatica-type symptoms, with pain originating in his right calf and progressing up his leg and into the lower right side of his back. It had progressively gotten worse over the previous two years, with the pain in his leg and lower back being exacerbated by walking only 200–300 yards (200–300m), at which point he had to stop because of the pain (mainly in his calf).

Medical History

This patient has been smoking about 60 cigarettes a day for the last 40 years. His blood pressure was tested to be 180/120. His right leg in particular appeared hairless and cold, with a reduction in his distal arterial pulses (posterior tibial and dorsalis pedis).

When I discuss this particular case with my students, the following medical conditions are considered to be the underlying causative factors for his symptoms:

- L5 or S1 referral (discogenic)
- Sacroiliac joint referral
- Lumbar facet joints
- Piriformis syndrome
- Sciatica
- Deep vein thrombosis

Again, let's consider the hypotheses for this patient. The patient denies any specific back or gluteal pain, and there is no history of any bending/twisting motions that might have aggravated the lumbar spine. As there is no apparent swelling/heat in his calf, we can also rule out a thrombosis.

My hypothesis for this diagnosis is that pain only comes on (initially) in his calf after walking 200–300 yards (200–300m), which entails an increase in demand for oxygen in his leg muscles. But there seems to be some difficulty in achieving this, resulting in an ischemic

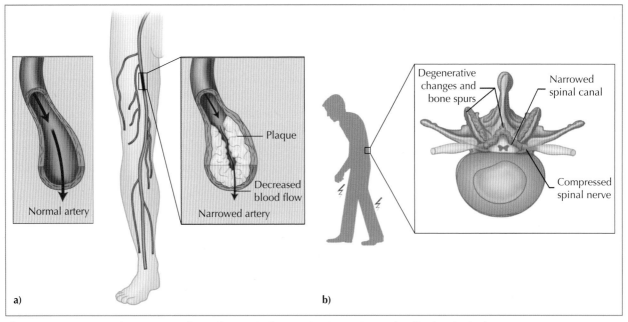

Figure 11.12: *Arteriosclerosis (a) and spinal stenosis (b), causing intermittent claudication in the legs.*

response (lack of blood to the tissues), subsequently causing an induction of pain in the associated soft tissues.

Let's think about the underlying causative factor here—my personal thought process was the following. The abdominal aorta splits into the iliac artery before becoming the femoral artery, which passes into the leg through the femoral triangle. In my consideration, he had an occlusion in the right iliac artery that was restricting the amount of blood going to his periphery, in particular to his lower limb. This condition is known as *intermittent claudication*, also referred to medically as *peripheral vascular disease* (PVD); it is no doubt mainly caused by thickening of the arteries, more commonly referred to as *arteriosclerosis* (Figure 11.12(a)).

This patient was recommended to visit his doctor, who referred him to a specialist; an arteriography was subsequently performed. The specialist diagnosed an occlusion in his right iliac artery, which resulted in surgical intervention. The patient has since given up smoking, and his blood pressure is continually being monitored.

Intermittent Claudication

Similar presenting conditions to those in Case Study 11.11 (leg pains), resulting from intermittent claudication, are also associated with *spinal stenosis*, which is a narrowing

of the spinal canal (Figure 11.12(b)) and classified as *neurological claudication*. However, as already explained, the diagnosis in Case Study 11.11 was *vascular claudication* due to thickening of the arteries (Figure 11.12(a)). The main difference is that in neurological claudication, the patient will need to flex their spine to open the spinal canal in order to ease the pressure, and thus reduce the symptoms, rather than just stopping walking.

Imagine the following situation: Malcolm and Doris, who are both 80 years old, are walking to the shops, but they both have to stop walking after 300 yards (300m) or so, because of the pain in their legs. Doris, on the one hand, just needs to stop walking for the pain in her legs to diminish, because she has vascular claudication, resulting from arteriosclerosis. Malcolm, on the other hand, has to bend forward to flex his spine in order to reduce the symptoms in his legs, because he has neurological claudication, caused by spinal stenosis.

Differential diagnosis – gallbladder, lung carcinoma, Virchow's lymph nodes

■ Conclusion

Hopefully, after reading about the medical conditions analyzed in the case studies in this chapter, my overall goal will have been met—namely, to make you more aware of some of the conditions that can give rise to patients with so-called "musculoskeletal presentations," and, in particular, with pain that presents itself in the neck, shoulder, thorax, lower back, and leg regions. The symptoms associated with underlying conditions that I discussed might be classified as *red flag conditions* and will require further investigation.

Remember that many patients will come to see a physical therapist first with any painful symptoms, rather than visit their primary care physician. We, as physical therapists, have a duty of care to all of the patients who walk through our clinic doors as regards their overall well-being. We need to know *when to treat* and, more importantly, *when not to treat* and, even more importantly, *when to refer to the medical profession*. That statement of "when to refer" has to be of the utmost priority, because it can simply be a life or death situation. I hope you bear that in mind that when the time comes!

There are, of course, a multitude of other conditions that I have not mentioned in this book that can refer pain via the neurological system and present as musculoskeletal pain. However, my focus is to try to make you aware of how some of the viscera actually refer pain to other structures within the musculoskeletal framework. With the correct questioning during the initial consultation and the appropriate orthopedic testing protocols, the practitioner can hopefully eliminate the musculoskeletal tissues as a source of a patient's presenting symptoms, especially if their symptoms cannot be reproduced during the physical therapy examination. It is then time to consider the possibility that the symptoms the patients are presenting with might actually be referred via the neurological system from an underlying condition of the viscera, rather than being simply musculoskeletal in origin.

12

Nerve Tension (Neurodynamic) Testing

The tests presented in this chapter are what I consider to be the most recognized and frequently used neural (also called *neurodynamic*) testing procedures found in any clinical setting. All of the described nerve tension tests (NTTs) can be utilized extremely effectively, as they are very easy to perform. The tests can be used either diagnostically to ascertain if a neural structure is involved in the patient's presenting symptoms, or therapeutically by incorporating them in treatment modalities. All of what I am about to describe can be implemented immediately by the physical therapist.

NTTs are classified as *neurodynamic* and can greatly assist the therapist in ascertaining if any components of the patient's neural structures are involved. Naturally, if a test is positive and the patient's presenting symptoms are exacerbated, one can confirm that the presence of their symptoms is connected in some way to the nervous system. The idea of neural tension testing is that the tests are designed to place stress on the peripheral neurological components of the upper and lower limbs.

Typically, the neural tests are performed on the asymptomatic side (non-painful side) first to elicit any possible symptoms/reactions, before the affected side is addressed. The procedure for each of the tests is carried out progressively, and each component is added in systematically, until the testing reproduces the patient's presenting symptoms (or does not, as the case may be). Even though these are generally classified as *diagnostic*

tests, the therapist can therapeutically modify the testing procedures and actually use these specific movements as part of a treatment process, to assist in desensitizing the nerves and ultimately reduce the symptoms.

Cautionary Note: One must be very careful when performing any of the following tests, especially on patients (or even on oneself) who visit the clinic for a consultation. The reason I say this is because, in the past, I have seen inexperienced therapists perform these procedures, some of which have brought on the patient's presenting symptoms quite quickly, which would naturally be regarded as a *positive test*. Utmost care must be taken at this critical point in the testing procedure, as it will be relatively easy to overstretch the tissues; these delicate neural structures can be very reactive if and when they are irritated. I have seen this happen in the clinic, where the patients were in a great deal more pain after the tests had finished, and I believe this to have happened because of the therapist's lack of experience.

To recap, if any type of pain or altered sensation—such as tingling or numbness—is experienced during any component of the testing position (and this includes the fine-tuning maneuvers for increased sensitization, which will be explained shortly), then the test will be classified as *positive*. Altered sensations are typically experienced in the areas of the neck, shoulder, arm, hand, and fingers (especially when the ULTTs are used), as well as in the lower limb, particularly the calf, foot, and toes.

The tests I will be discussing are:

1. Straight leg raise (SLR) test—Lasegue's sign (for the sciatic nerve)
2. Femoral nerve stretch—reverse Lasegue's sign (for the femoral nerve)
3. Opposite SLR (for sciatic symptoms)
4. Slump test
5. Upper limb tension tests (ULTTs)—median, ulnar, and radial nerves

■ 1. Straight Leg Raise (SLR) Test—Lasegue's Sign

I would say that most physical therapists will be familiar with Lasegue's sign, as this particular neural test is performed frequently in a clinical setting with patients whom one suspects have what are potentially herniated discs and are presenting with sciatic-type symptoms (sciatica). The test is named after Charles Lasegue, who first described it in 1864 as a way of increasing back pain when the straight leg is lifted into the air.

The patient will typically experience sciatic-type symptoms in their lower back and leg with passive hip flexion in the 30–70-degree range; this is suggestive of a lumbar spine disc condition, which tends to occur in the nerve roots between levels L4 and S1. If pain is felt below 30 degrees of hip flexion, this might indicate acute spinal symptoms, which can relate to many types of spinal condition, such as acute spondylolisthesis or even tumors. Pain after 70 degrees of flexion is probably due to tightness of the hamstrings.

Technique

- Instruct the patient to adopt a supine position.
- Test each leg, but initially the normal leg (asymptomatic).
- Take control of the patient's lower limb.
- Slowly internally rotate the patient's leg and then lift it into hip flexion.
- If the patient experiences sciatic or back pain between 30 and 70 degrees, this is classified as a *positive test* (Figure 12.1).

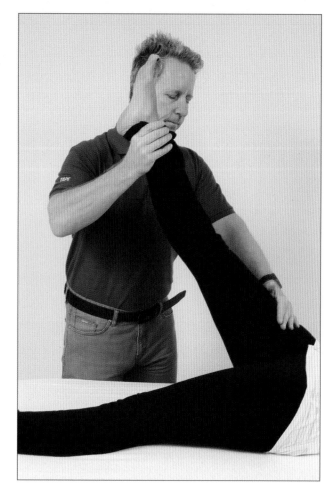

Figure 12.1: *Straight leg raise (SLR) test: sciatic pain is indicated at 50 degrees of hip flexion.*

Summary of the test for Lasegue's sign:

1. Patient supine.
2. Hip internal rotation.
3. Hip flexion 30–70 degrees.

Variations of the SLR Test

We can add some fine-tuning variations to the standard SLR test in order to increase the sensitizations; these variations are potentially more effective, as they increase the specificity to the neural structures being tested.

SLR Test Combined with Ankle Dorsiflexion

In the first of the extra tests, the standard SLR test is initially performed to see if the patient experiences increased neurological symptoms, especially in the posterior part of the lower leg and foot. After the initial motion, the therapist slowly brings them out of the standard SLR position while slowly passively *dorsiflexing* the ankle joint, as this will stretch the *tibial* component of the sciatic nerve (Figure 12.2).

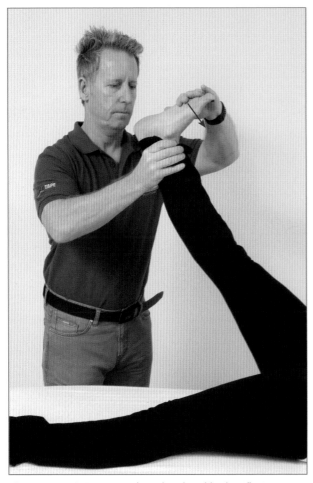

Figure 12.2: *SLR test combined with ankle dorsiflexion.*

SLR Test Combined with Ankle Plantar Flexion and Inversion

The second variation is similar to the first, but this time, and especially if the patient experiences symptoms in the anterior surface of the lower limb and dorsal foot, we slowly bring them out of the standard SLR position while slowly passively *plantar flexing* and then *inverting* the ankle joint, as this will stretch the *common fibular* component of the sciatic nerve (Figure 12.3).

 **Straight leg raise test (SLR)**

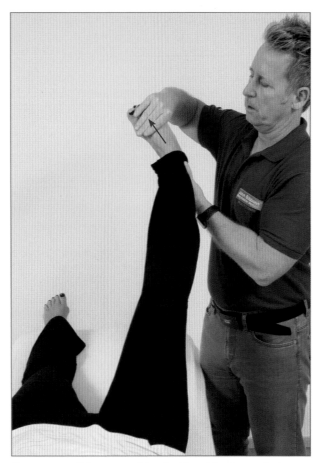

Figure 12.3: *SLR test combined with ankle plantar flexion and inversion.*

SLR Test Combined with Cervical Flexion

The third option is again from the Lasegue position, but this time patient is asked to slowly bring their chin to their chest while they are experiencing the leg symptoms. If including the flexion of the cervical spine exacerbates the symptoms in their leg, then this is another positive test for a disc condition, as cervical flexion stretches the dura matter of the spinal cord (Figure 12.4).

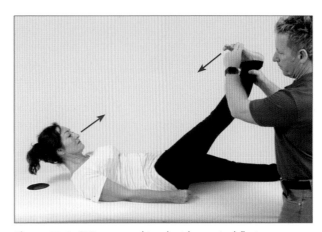

Figure 12.4: *SLR test combined with cervical flexion.*

■ 2. Femoral Nerve Stretch—Reverse Lasegue's Sign

The reverse Lasegue's sign is useful for identifying the involvement of the femoral nerve, where typically the patient will have neurological symptoms in the anterior thigh area of their quadriceps, as shown in Figure 12.5.

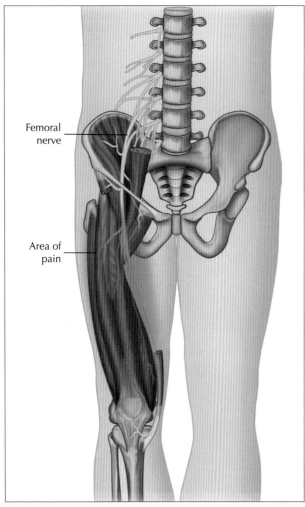

Figure 12.5: *Femoral nerve pain located in the anterior thigh.*

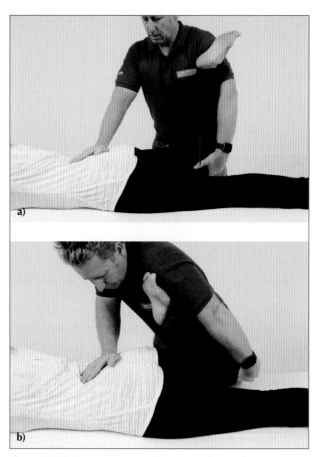

Figure 12.6: *Reverse Lasegue's sign: (a) femoral nerve stretch; (b) combined knee flexion and hip extension.*

Summary of the test for reverse Lasegue's sign:

1. Patient prone.
2. Knee flexion.
3. Hip extension.

 **Femoral nerve testing**

Technique

- Instruct the patient to adopt a prone position.
- First, apply a simple stretch to the patient's quadriceps by flexing their knee, as shown in Figure 12.6(a).
- Second, maintain the position of knee flexion and then slowly extend the patient's hip joint.
- If this maneuver exacerbates the symptoms, this is indicative of a positive test for femoral nerve pain (Figure 12.6(b)).

■ 3. Opposite SLR Test—Sciatic Symptoms

I consider the opposite SLR test to be effective for detecting a potential disc condition, even though it is not used very often by physical therapists. Imagine your patient has what you believe to be neurological pain in the back of their *left* leg. If you were to perform the SLR test on their *right* leg (Figure 12.7), or even a simple hamstring

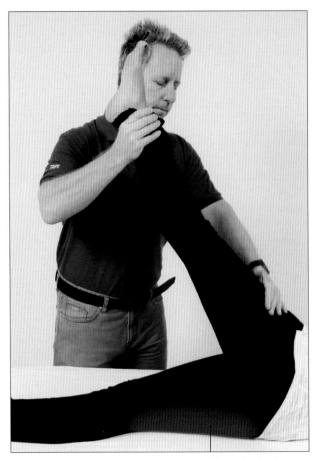

Figure 12.7: *Opposite SLR test – pain is felt in the back of the left leg.*

- If the pain is in the patient's right leg, test their asymptomatic side first: ask them to extend their left knee, and then combine this with dorsiflexion of their left ankle.
- Ask the patient to lean forward (thoracic flexion), and to finally slump their body by bringing their chin to their chest.
- Repeat the procedure on the patient's painful side.
- If the patient has true sciatic pain, most of these added motions will increase the patient's symptoms.

Summary of the slump test:

1. Patient seated with hands behind back.
2. Knee extension.
3. Ankle dorsiflexion.
4. Thoracic flexion.
5. Cervical flexion.

 Slump test

stretch on their right side, then the patient might actually feel the symptoms increase in the *opposite* leg (left leg in this case). This test is believed to be indicative of a lower lumbar disc condition.

■ 4. Slump Test

The slump test is probably one of the most popular procedures for identifying sciatic nerve pain. The test is typically done in stages (see below), although I modify the procedure (compared with how it was initially shown to me) for my own use, because I believe all the components of the test can be incorporated into one simple maneuver.

Technique

- Instruct the patient to sit upright on a couch with their hands behind their back and their legs hanging off the edge (Figure 12.8(a)–(d)).

■ 5. Upper Limb Tension Tests

It might sound strange to hear this, but the following techniques were not specifically taught to me during my five-year osteopathy program. However, I did my initial training many years ago, and I have subsequently learned a lot of techniques since then, so I now consider myself proficient in what I am about to describe.

If possible, we could try to specify tests for the individual peripheral nerves from the brachial plexus, as we are basically looking for a cervical radiculopathy. The nerves of concern in this text are the median, ulnar, and radial nerves. These particular tests were first described by Elvey (1994), and needless to say are referred to as the *Elvey tests*. They are also known as the *brachial plexus tension tests*, but, in clinical practice, the most common term used is *upper limb tension tests* (ULTTs).

The specific nerve we will be testing is identified in the names of the tests presented below; if we do happen to find a positive result, we can then utilize these testing procedures to mobilize the entrapped nerve.

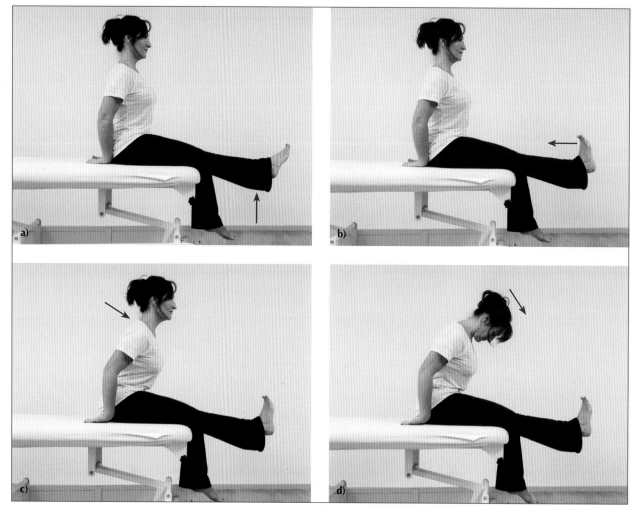

Figure 12.8: *Slump test: (a) patient is seated with hands behind back and knee extended; (b) patient dorsiflexes their ankle; (c) thoracic flexion is added; (d) the last component, cervical flexion, is added.*

ULTT—Median Nerve

- Instruct the patient to adopt a supine position.
- Initially apply shoulder girdle depression to the patient, then externally rotate and abduct their shoulder to 90 degrees (Figure 12.9(a)–(b)).
- Next, add in wrist and finger extension (Figure 12.9(c)).
- From this position, slowly extend the patient's elbow, making sure that their forearm is in supination (Figure 12.9(d)).
- Finally, ask the patient to side bend their neck to the opposite side (Figure 12.9(e)).
- If the symptoms in the arm are exacerbated, it can be assumed that the median nerve is involved.

Summary of the ULTT of the median nerve:

1. Patient supine.
2. Shoulder girdle depression.
3. External rotation of shoulder.
4. Shoulder abduction to 90 degrees.
5. Wrist and finger extension.
6. Elbow extension.
7. Lateral flexion of cervical spine.

ULTT – median nerve

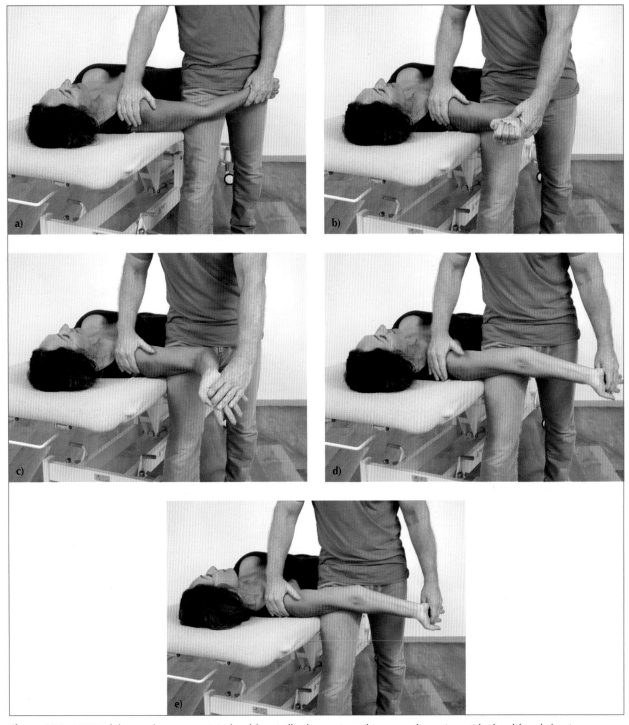

Figure 12.9: *ULTT of the median nerve: (a) shoulder girdle depression; (b) external rotation with shoulder abduction to 90 degrees; (c) wrist and finger extension; (d) elbow extension; (e) lateral flexion of cervical spine.*

ULTT—Ulnar Nerve

- Instruct the patient to adopt a supine position.
- Initially apply shoulder girdle depression to the patient, externally rotate their shoulder, and then slowly flex their elbow and abduct their shoulder to 90 degrees (Figure 12.10(a)–(c)).

- Next, slowly extend the patient's wrist and fingers, then add in forearm pronation (Figure 12.10(d)–(e)).
- From this position, slowly flex their elbow and abduct their shoulder past 90 degrees (Figure 12.10(f)).
- Finally, ask the patient to side bend their neck to the opposite side (Figure 12.10(g)).
- If the symptoms in the arm are exacerbated, it can be assumed that the ulnar nerve is involved.

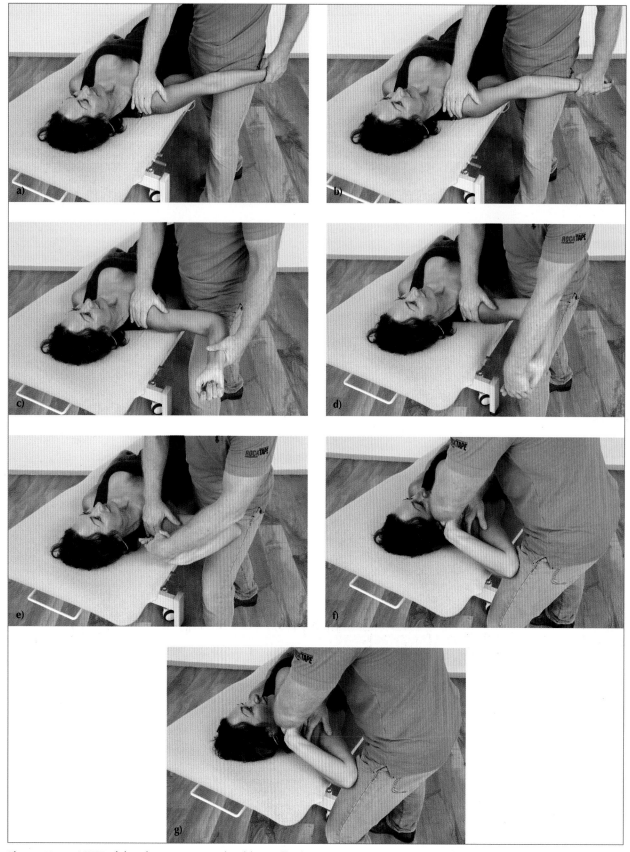

Figure 12.10: *ULTT of the ulnar nerve: (a) shoulder girdle depression; (b) external rotation of shoulder; (c) elbow flexion with shoulder abduction to 90 degrees; (d) wrist and finger extension; (e) pronation of forearm; (f) elbow flexion and shoulder abduction past 90 degrees; (g) lateral flexion of cervical spine.*

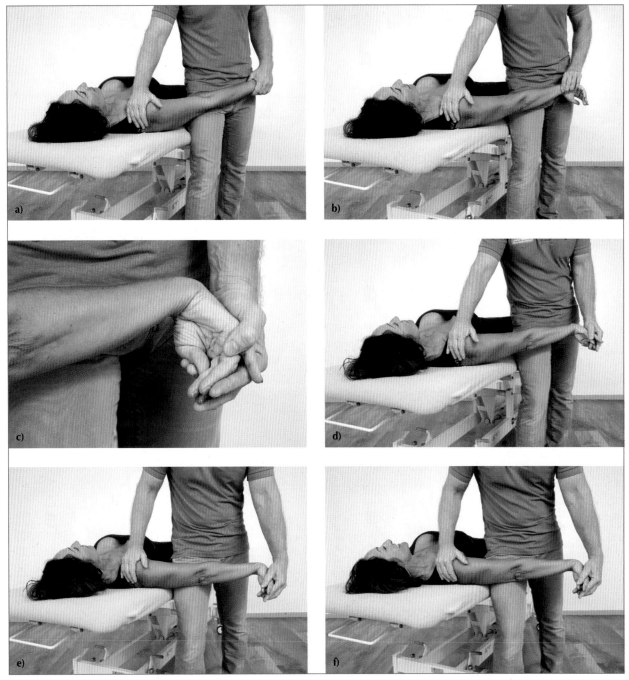

Figure 12.11: *ULTT of the radial nerve: (a) shoulder girdle depression; (b) internal rotation of arm; (c) wrist, finger, and thumb flexion; (d) ulnar deviation; (e) shoulder abduction to 70–90 degrees; (f) lateral flexion of cervical spine.*

Summary of the ULTT of the ulnar nerve:

1. Patient supine.
2. Shoulder girdle depression.
3. External rotation of shoulder.
4. Elbow flexion and shoulder abduction to 90 degrees.
5. Wrist and finger extension.
6. Pronation of forearm.
7. Elbow flexion past 90 degrees.
8. Shoulder abduction past 90 degrees.
9. Lateral flexion of cervical spine.

ULTT – ulnar nerve

ULTT—Radial Nerve

- Instruct the patient to adopt a supine position.
- Initially apply shoulder girdle depression to the patient, then take the patient's arm into full internal rotation (Figure 12.11(a)–(b)).
- Next, slowly flex the patient's wrist, fingers, and finally thumb, and add in ulnar deviation to the wrist (Figure 12.11(c)–(d)).
- From this position, abduct the patient's shoulder to around 70–90 degrees (Figure 12.11(e)).
- Finally, ask the patient to side bend their head to the opposite side (Figure 12.11(f)).
- If the symptoms in the arm are exacerbated, it can be assumed that the radial nerve is involved.

Summary of the ULTT of the radial nerve:

1. Patient supine.
2. Shoulder girdle depression.
3. Internal rotation of the arm.
4. Wrist, finger, and thumb flexion.
5. Ulnar deviation of wrist.
6. Shoulder abduction to 70–90 degrees.
7. Lateral flexion of cervical spine.

ULTT – radial nerve

Conclusion

I personally believe that all therapists involved in assessing and subsequently treating or referring patients should have at least the basic skills and understanding of appropriately ascertaining whether the peripheral nervous system is functioning correctly.

Let me give you an example. Many soft-tissue (massage) therapists will never have been taught anything related to the nervous system (especially in the UK); this is mainly a shortcoming of the training curriculum, which is a shame but a relatively normal state of affairs, especially with short intensive courses. However, at some point in their careers, one of these massage therapists will come across a patient presenting with, let's say, shoulder and arm pain, and this may be combined with a presentation of some weakness in their arm/s when they perform daily tasks. The therapist will probably treat the area of pain (possible symptoms), rather than trying to find out which structures are actually responsible for causing the patient's presenting symptoms.

I hope that after reading this book you will realize that the patient above could have prolapsed a cervical disc and that the herniation is causing pressure on the exiting C5 nerve root, possibly explaining why they have weakness in lifting their arm and subsequent pain in the shoulder area. If one follows a comprehensive assessment procedure through the use of, for example, a simple reflex (patella) hammer, in combination with muscle strength testing (myotome testing) and sensory testing by means of the dermatomes, not forgetting the essential specific questioning during the initial consultation, one might come up with a realistic hypothesis as to what is causing the patient's painful symptoms.

Once the therapist has all this extra knowledge, they can then decide on the best cause of action, which in actuality may well be a referral to a medical doctor for further investigation, such as an MRI scan. However, if the therapist is both confident and competent, they might decide to treat the patient themselves before they refer them, if necessary, to another practitioner. They will then at least gain a better understanding of where the source of the pain is (e.g., cervical), rather than simply rubbing where it hurts (e.g., shoulder and arm) … and with the correct treatment strategies, the patient's presenting symptoms might actually start to reduce. Naturally, if the symptoms persist, a referral would then be the recommended course of action.

My goal was to write a different type of book on nerves— one where therapists (mainly) would actually understand the subject being discussed, but, more importantly, enjoy what it is they are reading and be able to retain some of what they have read, because I was able to make it interesting for them. That is my main mission with all the books I write: I want people to experience the excitement and anticipation of reading the text and derive actual pleasure from what I have written. If they don't, what would be the point of it all? My books would otherwise live on the owners' bookshelves like all the rest of their books and never actually get read. Sadly, the only thing that would happen to the books is they would collect dust, just like a vintage bottle of wine … now and again we look at the bottle, blow the dust off, and place it back without actually sampling its contents. I will leave that thought with you!

Bibliography

Adson, A.W., and Coffey, J.R. 1927. "Cervical rib: A method of anterior approach for relief of symptoms by division of the scalenus anticus," *Ann Surg* 85: 839–857.

Anekstein, Y., Blecher, R., Smorgick, Y., et al. 2012. "What is the best way to apply the Spurling test for cervical radiculopathy," *Clin Orthop Relat Res* 470(9): 2566–2572.

Boyling, J.D., and Palastanga, N. (eds) 1994. *Grieve's Modern Manual Therapy: The Vertebral Column*, 2nd edn, Edinburgh: Churchill Livingstone.

Dyck, P.J., Karnes, J., O'Brien, P., et al. 1984. "Spatial pattern of nerve fibre abnormality indicative of pathologic mechanism," *Am J Pathol* 117(2): 225–238.

Elvey, R.L. 1994. "The investigation of arm pain," in Boyling and Palastanga (1994).

Esene, I.N., Meher, A., Elzoghby, M.A., et al. 2012. "Diagnostic performance of the medial hamstring reflex in L5 radiculopathy," *Surg Neurol Int* 3: 104.

Gillard, J., Perez-Cousin, M., Hachulla, E., et al. 2001. "Diagnosing thoracic outlet syndrome: Contribution of provocation tests, ultrasonography, electrophysiology, and helical computed tomography in 48 patients," *Joint Bone Spine* 68: 416–424.

Malanga, G.A., and Nadler, S.F. 2006. *Musculoskeletal Physical Examination: An Evidence-based Approach*, Philadelphia: Mosby, 50–51.

Naffziger, H.C., and Grant, W.T. 1938. "Neuritis of the brachial plexus mechanical in origin: The scalene syndrome," *Surg Gynecol Obstet* 67: 722.

Novak, C.B., and Mackinnon, S.E. 1996. "Thoracic outlet syndrome," *Occupat Disord Manag* 27(4): 747–762.

Plewa, M.C., and Delinger, M. 1998. "The false positive rate of thoracic outlet syndrome shoulder maneuvers in healthy individuals," *Acad Emerg Med* 5: 337–342.

Rezzouk, J., Uzel, M., Lavignolle, B., et al. 2004. "Does the motor branch of the long head of the triceps brachii arise from the radial nerve?," *Surg Radiol Anat* 26(6): 459–461.

Rob, C.G., and Standeven, A. 1958. "Arterial occlusion complicating thoracic outlet compression syndrome," *Br Med J* 2: 709–712.

Roos, D. 1996. "Historical perspectives and anatomic considerations: Thoracic outlet syndrome," *Semin Thorac Cardiovasc Surg* 8(2): 183–189.

Smith, D.R., Kobrine, A.I., and Rizzoli, H.V. 1977. "Absence of autoregulation in peripheral nerve blood flow," *J Neurol Sci* 33: 347–352.

Spurling, R.S., and Scoville, W.B. 1944. "Lateral rupture of the cervical intervertebral discs: A common cause of shoulder and arm pain," *Surg Gynecol Obstet* 78: 350–358.

Umphred, D.A. (ed.) 2001. *Neurological Rehabilitation*, 4th edn, St Louis: Mosby.

Umphred, D.A., Byl, N., Lazaro, R.T., and Roller, M. 2001. "Interventions for neurological disabilities," in Umphred (2001), 56–134.

Vanti, C., Natalini, L., Romeo, A., et al. 2007. "Conservative treatment of thoracic outlet syndrome: A review of the literature," *Eura Medicophys* 43: 55–70.

Appendix

Table A.1: List of cranial nerves.

Number	Name of nerve	Nerve type	Function
I	Olfactory	Sensory	Smell
II	Optic	Sensory	Vision
III	Oculomotor	Motor	Most eye movement control
IV	Trochlear	Motor	Eye movement coordination (superior oblique muscle)
V	Trigeminal	Mixed	Face and mouth sensation, muscles of mastication control
VI	Abducens	Motor	Eye abduction (lateral rectus muscle)
VII	Facial	Mixed	Muscles of facial expression, lacrimal and salivary glands (taste)
VIII	Vestibulocochlear	Sensory	Hearing and balance
IX	Glossopharyngeal	Mixed	Gag reflex, sense of taste and serve the pharynx for swallowing
X	Vagus	Mixed	Gag reflex, control of heart, parasympathetic innervation of muscles of viscera
XI	Accessory	Motor	Shoulder shrugging and movement of neck
XII	Hypoglossal	Motor	Swallowing, speech, movement of tongue

Table A.2: Differences between upper and lower motor neuron lesions.

UMN lesion symptoms	LMN lesion symptoms
Hyperreflexia	Hyporeflexia
Hypertonicity	Hypotonicity
Spasticity	Flaccid paralysis
Babinski reflex positive	Babinski reflex negative
Clonus present	Fasciculation and fibrillation

Table A.3: Specific reflexes for the upper and lower limbs.

Area tested for reflex	Corresponding spinal level
Biceps tendon	C5
Brachioradialis (forearm)	C6
Triceps (elbow)	C7
Adductors	L3
Patellar tendon	L4
Medial hamstrings	L5
Achilles tendon	S1
Plantar (foot)	S1
External anal sphincter	S3/S4
Babinski (plantar)	Upper motor neuron (CNS)

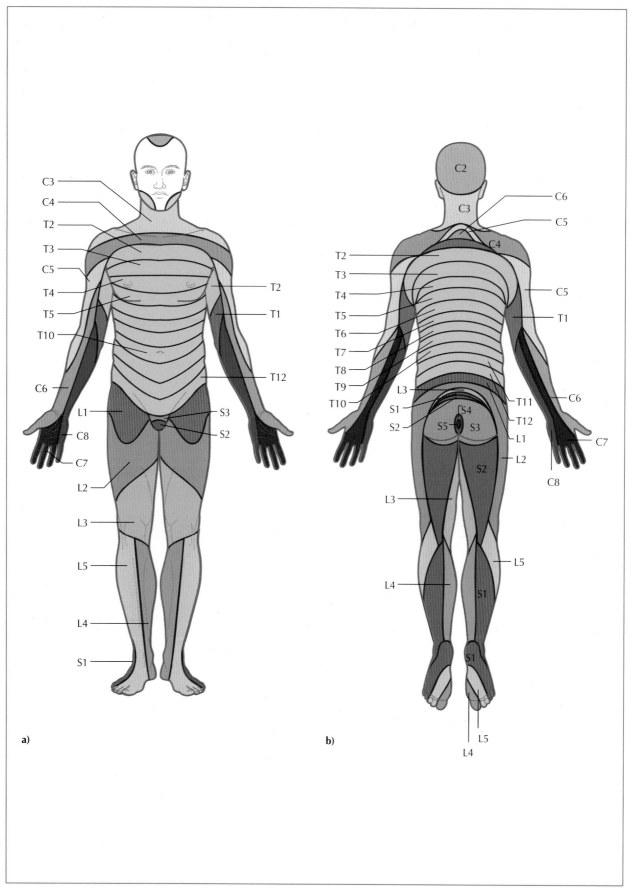

Figure A.1: *Map of the dermatomes of the body: (a) anterior and (b) posterior views.*

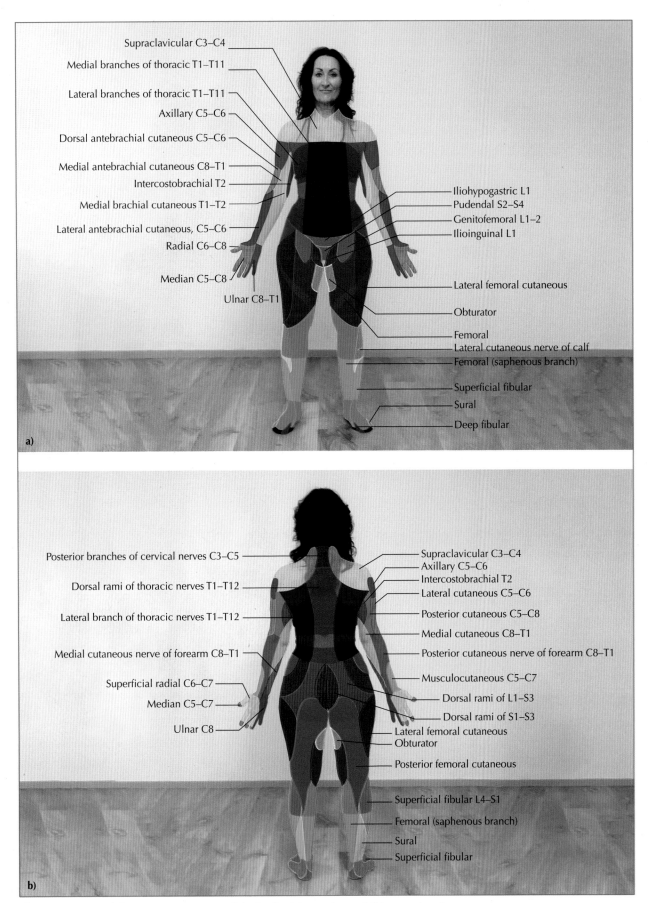

Supraclavicular C3–C4

Medial branches of thoracic T1–T11

Lateral branches of thoracic T1–T11

Axillary C5–C6

Dorsal antebrachial cutaneous C5–C6

Medial antebrachial cutaneous C8–T1

Intercostobrachial T2

Medial brachial cutaneous T1–T2

Lateral antebrachial cutaneous, C5–C6

Radial C6–C8

Median C5–C8

Ulnar C8–T1

Iliohypogastric L1
Pudendal S2–S4
Genitofemoral L1–2
Ilioinguinal L1

Lateral femoral cutaneous

Obturator

Femoral

Lateral cutaneous nerve of calf

Femoral (saphenous branch)

Superficial fibular

Sural

Deep fibular

a)

Posterior branches of cervical nerves C3–C5

Dorsal rami of thoracic nerves T1–T12

Lateral branch of thoracic nerves T1–T12

Medial cutaneous nerve of forearm C8–T1

Superficial radial C6–C7

Median C5–C7

Ulnar C8

Supraclavicular C3–C4
Axillary C5–C6
Intercostobrachial T2
Lateral cutaneous C5–C6
Posterior cutaneous C5–C8
Medial cutaneous C8–T1
Posterior cutaneous nerve of forearm C8–T1
Musculocutaneous C5–C7
Dorsal rami of L1–S3
Dorsal rami of S1–S3
Lateral femoral cutaneous
Obturator
Posterior femoral cutaneous
Superficial fibular L4–S1
Femoral (saphenous branch)
Sural
Superficial fibular

b)

Figure A.2: *Map of the cutaneous nerves of the body: (a) anterior and (b) posterior views.*

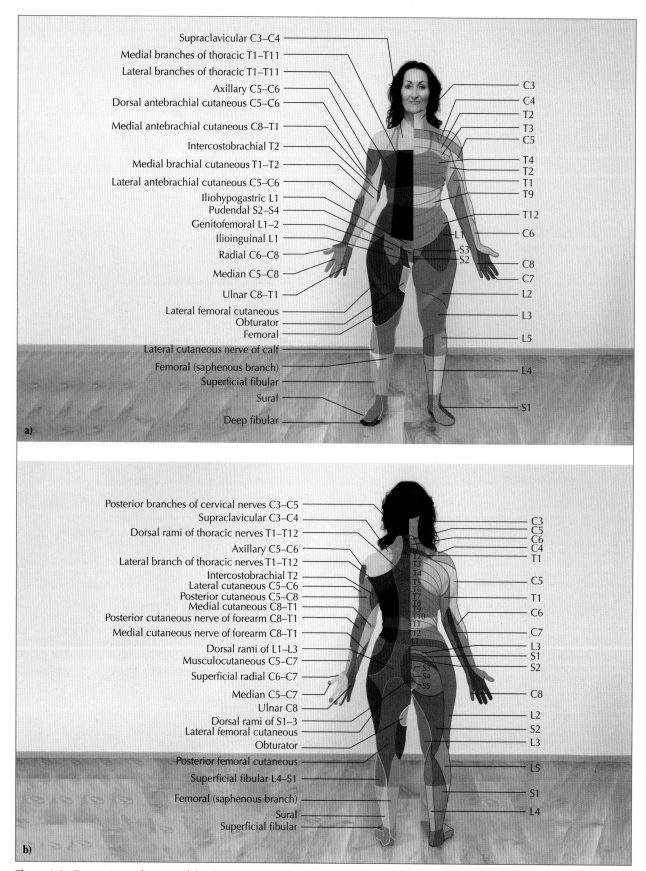

Figure A.3: *Comparison of a map of the dermatomes and the cutaneous nerves of the body: (a) anterior and (b) posterior views.*

Table A.4: A dermatome versus a cutaneous nerve.

Dermatome	Cutaneous nerve
A *dermatome* is a sensory region located on the body that is supplied by a single spinal nerve root.	*Cutaneous innervation* is a localized sensory region of the skin that is innervated by a specific cutaneous nerve.

Table A.5: Map of the dermatomes of the upper body.

Dermatome location—upper body	Spinal level
Occipital protuberance and posterior neck	C2
Anterior neck and supraclavicular fossa	C3
Supraclavicular fossa and acromioclavicular joint	C4
Infraclavicular area and across upper limb to above elbow	C5
Lateral forearm and thumb	C6
Middle finger	C7
Little finger	C8
Medial forearm	T1

Table A.6: Map of the dermatomes of the thoracic spine.

Dermatome location—thoracic spine	Spinal level
Medial forearm	T1
Medial upper arm and axilla	T2
Superior to nipple line	T3
Level of nipple line	T4
Superior to xiphoid process	T5
Level of xiphoid process	T6
Inferior to xiphoid process	T7
Halfway between xiphoid process and umbilicus	T8
Superior to umbilicus	T9
Level of umbilicus	T10
Inferior to umbilicus	T11
Suprapubic area, level with iliac crest	T12

Table A.7: Map of the dermatomes of the lower body.

Dermatome location—lower body	Spinal level
Below inguinal ligament, groin	L1
Upper thigh	L2
Anterior thigh to knee	L3
Medial aspect of lower leg and medial malleolus	L4
Lateral aspect of lower leg, dorsum of foot and toes 1–4	L5
Lateral aspect of foot and little toe, lateral malleolus, heel, and majority of sole of foot	S1
Posterior aspect of thigh and popliteal fossa	S2
Concentric rings around anus (we sit on S3), area of ischial tuberosity	S3
Skin over perianal area and genitals	S4
Skin next to anus as well as perianal area	S5

Note: I mentioned the lack of map consistency earlier, and I consider it an interesting peculiarity in one respect that some dermatome maps show the L5 dermatome covering the great toe (hallux), while others show the L4 dermatome covering that particular area. Just bear in mind, therefore, that variations do exist, and so it is difficult to say which one is actually correct.

Table A.8: Grading system for the myotomes.

0	No muscle contraction is visible
1	Muscle contraction is visible but there is no movement of the joint
2	Active joint movement is possible with gravity eliminated
3	Movement can overcome gravity but not resistance from the examiner
4	The muscle group can overcome gravity and move against some resistance from the examiner
5	Full and normal power against resistance

Table A.9: Map of the myotomes of the upper limb.

Myotome location—upper limb	Spinal level
Cervical flexion/extension	C1/C2
Cervical lateral flexion	C3
Shoulder elevation	C4
Shoulder abduction and elbow flexion	C5
Elbow flexion and wrist extension	C6
Elbow extension, wrist flexion, and finger extension	C7
Finger flexion	C8
Finger abduction and adduction	T1

Table A.10: Map of the myotomes of the lower limb.

Myotome location—lower limb	Spinal level
Hip flexion	L2
Knee extension	L3
Ankle dorsiflexion	L4
Great toe (hallux) extension	L5
Ankle plantar flexion/eversion and hip extension	S1
Knee flexion	S2

Index